The Journal of a
Teenage Pregnancy

The Journal
of a teenage pregnancy

by Erin Elias

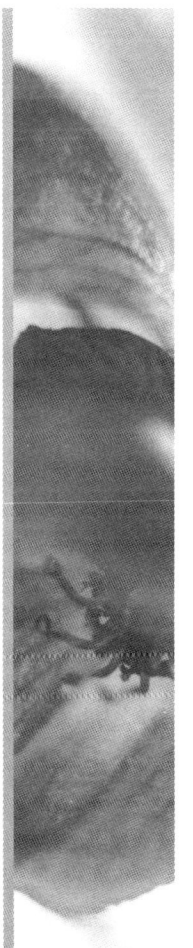

Guardian
BOOKS

Belleville, Ontario, Canada

First Printing: February 2004
Second Printing: March 2007
Third Printing: May 2009

National Library of Canada Cataloguing in Publication
Elias, Erin, 1982-
    The journal of a teenage pregnancy / Erin Elias.
Includes bibliographical references.
ISBN 978-1-55306-774-0
    1. Elias, Erin, 1982- --Diaries. 2. Teenage pregnancy. 3. Teenage mothers--Diaries. 4. Unmarried mothers--Diaries. I. Title.
HQ759.4.E44 2004   306.874'3'092   C2003-907506-0

**For more information or
to order additional copies, please contact:**

erindelias@hotmail.com

Guardian Books is an imprint of *Essence Publishing,* a Christian Book Publisher dedicated to furthering the work of Christ through the written word For more information, contact:
20 Hanna Court, Belleville, Ontario, Canada K8P 5J2
Phone: 1-800-238-6376 • Fax: (613) 962-3055
E-mail: info@essence-publishing.com
Web site: www.essence-publishing.com

Dedication

To every girl who has stared at a positive pregnancy test in fear,
and to my husband, without whom I never would have made it.

Prologue

I look back on those six months of my life now, two years after it happened, and it looks like a big, black hole—a dark ages, of sorts—in the timeline of my life. I say "six months" because I found out about it two months after it started and it ended a month before it was supposed to. Sometimes I'm really thankful that I didn't know for the full nine months. Being pregnant when you are eighteen just isn't something that you really remember fondly.

Yes, I was only eighteen. My life was so simple at the time. I lived in Winnipeg with two of my friends during the week and went home to my parents' for weekends. The three of us had a little basement apartment. Teresa was my roommate from high school and Karen was a former co-worker who had nowhere else to go. I invited her to live with us while she sorted her life out. I was working at a cats-only vet clinic, a short bike ride from our apartment. I had graduated from college with a "veterinary hospital office assistant" diploma, and that's the job I was doing—well, reception; same thing. I had only been working there for about a month. But it was a great job. My boss was so friendly and caring, I came to think of her as a second mother. My co-workers were all females who understood and sympathized without judging.

And there was my boyfriend. Phill and I had been dating for two and a half years. We were good Christian teens from good Christian homes and had both graduated from a good Christian school. I don't know what was wrong with us. I guess we were young and stupid and felt, like most young people, that we were invincible. And I guess we had just been dating too long. When we first started going out, our classmates made fun of us because we were too shy to even hold hands for the first two weeks! It took us months before we kissed for the first time. But things kept progressing after that, until eventually we were comfortable doing almost anything, and then we found ourselves doing everything.

I once heard it explained like this: if you put a frog in a pot of boiling water, it will immediately jump out. But if you put that same frog in a pot of cold water and then slowly heat it up on the stove, it will boil to death because it won't realize how hot it's getting. I thought the explanation was cheesy at the time, but now I know how true it is.

I suppose it was a combination of a lot of things, but the fact of the matter was that we were having sex. We knew it was wrong. We didn't want to keep doing it. We tried, and vowed many times, to stop. But once you cross that line, it's almost like there's no turning back.

I saw my Christian life start to crumble. I couldn't pray any more. Why would God listen? I was doing something I knew was so wrong, and yet, no matter how many times I told Him that I would stop, I kept on doing it. I quit asking for help. I felt guilty. I felt I couldn't ask for help. Why would God want to help me? I was such a failure.

And then one day my daily journal entries turned from normal, simple life to complicated, hard life. I was pregnant. It was scary, shocking, hopeless. It felt like it was the end of my life. And that's why I'm sharing it with you. When I was feeling all those things, I longed for direction. I felt so alone. I wanted to read about someone else going through the same thing. I didn't want to make another mistake.

So if you are the one feeling scared, hopeless, and lost, please read on. What you will find is my journal, kept during the last six months of my pregnancy. It is an honest, unchanged account of what I thought and felt during that dark time. I know I made mistakes and thought things I shouldn't have, but I make no apologies for including them. This is exactly how it was. I also know that I had a very hard time trusting the Lord Jesus and waiting on Him. But, in the end, I learned that very important lesson.

I hope my experiences will leave you feeling a little less alone, a little more hopeful. I hope you will recognize that, no matter how bad things get, there is always hope, and that Jesus does not abandon us. I don't plan to give you all the answers or tell you what you should do. Every situation is different, and one solution doesn't fix everyone's problems. But when you are through reading this journal, perhaps you will know which mistakes not to make. I'm positive that you will know that God cares about you and that He can do anything you think is impossible. If you put your hope in Him, He will never disappoint you.

Remembering mine affliction and my misery, the wormwood and the gall. My soul hath them still in remembrance, and is humbled in me. This I recall to my mind, therefore have I hope. It is of the LORD's mercies that we are not consumed, because his compassions fail not. They are new every morning: great is thy faithfulness. The LORD is my portion, saith my soul; therefore will I hope in him. The LORD is good unto them that wait for him, to the soul that seeketh him. It is good that a man should both hope and quietly wait for the salvation of the LORD. (Lamentations 3:19-26).

July

Dear Journal,

A couple of people have suggested to me that I may be stressed out. Work has been especially bad the last couple of days. I've worked two and a half hours of overtime, we have so many cats in boarding that it takes forever to clean all their cages, the vet that we have working right now keeps making the clients mad and then to top it all off, our partner clinic phoned and reemed me out for sending clients to them! I only did it because our vet told me to. Plus, we had to do month-end today, which always takes a long time.

What else is worrying me? Phill, pregnancy, not enough sleep, friends...no wonder my period won't come. I can't eat and my stomach hurts all the time. The long weekend coming up sounds so good but it looks like it won't be relaxing either.

Dear Journal

I'm so thankful I only had to work until noon today. Then I picked up a sub for lunch and went for a manicure and pedicure. It was very relaxing. When I got home I did my laundry and slept for an hour.

I'm getting really concerned about my period. Today is the 50th day of my cycle. I'm usually irregular but never this bad. I've been having cramps for two weeks and still nothing. But I don't think I'm pregnant because I would be having more symptoms if I was. Phill is very worried. I keep trying to reassure him but I'm getting a little worried myself. Seven weeks is a little long already. One of these days we're going to have to smarten up. I can't live like this, never knowing if the next period is going to come. But I just don't trust myself. I always fail.

Dear Journal

I'm getting very nervous about what's happening to me. Tomorrow it will be eight weeks since my last period. I think I've been having PMS for the last three weeks, but nothing is happening. Isn't missing a period the first clue that you're pregnant?

Dear Journal,

I don't believe this is happening. My boyfriend, Phill, called me at work yesterday. He had been reading up on the symptoms of pregnancy on the internet and didn't like what he read. I've had some of the symptoms he read about. But I haven't had all of them—no nausea, morning sickness, or cravings. And I was still having normal PMS cramps up until yesterday morning. Suddenly they've stopped, too. We tried to figure out what's happened since my last period and everything seems to be fine. We don't think we've had sex this past month.

But this morning I walked to the drugstore and picked up a home pregnancy test just to be sure. That was nerve-racking enough, never mind actually doing the test! I was so nervous walking into that drugstore, I couldn't look the cashier in the eye. I just hoped that she wouldn't care or look at me funny. Once she had put it in a bag and I had paid for it, I left and vowed never to go there again. I came home and hid it in my desk drawer so my roommates wouldn't see it. I think I'll do it tonight after they both leave. Karen is going out with her boyfriend and Teresa has to work, so I will be free to do it without having to hide it from them.

I'm really scared! If I do turn out to be pregnant, what will I do? I don't think I could face anyone I know. I've always been a "good girl," and no one will expect this from me. I think a lot of people who find out will want to tell me exactly what they think of me. The thing is, I know what we've been doing is stupid. I feel guilty enough already without everyone else telling me I should be.

I keep wanting to pray for mercy, but I don't feel as though I can. This is exactly what I deserve. Why would I expect God to deliver me from a deserving punishment? I don't know what to do. How am I going to tell Phill? I don't know how he's going to react. Even worse, how will I tell Mom and Dad? How will I go to church, knowing what everyone will think of me?

I've been crying a lot, just thinking about the awful possibilities. What made me cry most was when, last night on the phone, I asked Phill if this in any way would wreck our relationship. He immediately said no, it wouldn't. He told me that he loves me very much and he wants to take care of me. That means more to me than anything else.

If I do end up being pregnant, I would really like to consider giving the baby up for adoption. Of course, I'll ask Phill if he agrees before I decide, but I don't see how I could keep it. It would complicate my life to no end. I don't know where I would live or how I would pay for it. I don't think I could have a baby and work at the same time. Phill still wants to go to university for two years, and I can't quit working. I just wonder how hard adoption would be. I guess we'll find out after I do the test tonight if we have to worry about any of these things. I have to get ready to go to work now.

My Dear Journal,

In a few months, you and Phill may be the only ones I can talk to ever again. I just did the test and it came up positive. I locked myself in the bathroom and started filling the bathtub with hot water; then I did it. While I was waiting for the result to come up, I couldn't even bear to peek at the test stick to see what it was doing. I was so nervous. Finally, when the time was up, I made myself look. Those two pink lines were staring me in the face: a positive result. My heart started pounding. I tossed the test in the garbage and got in the tub. My mind was racing. I kept looking at my distorted reflection in the chrome piece under the faucet, trying to imagine what I would look like with a big belly.

Maybe we were just in denial, but we actually felt pretty confident that the test would be negative. And now I'm pregnant. It's so hard to believe, to wrap my mind around. I guess the first thing I need to do is call Phill. I'll also have to tell my boss, Caroline, at the clinic so that I don't have to assist with x-raying any pets. It's part of my job, but I have to protect the baby.

When am I going to tell Mom and Dad and the rest of my family? In nine months, what on earth am I going to do? I guess I need to see a doctor now. Could the test have been screwed up? The leaflet said only an out-of-uterus pregnancy could affect the results. What is Phill going to do? Will we get married? I guess not, if we don't keep the baby. I still can't believe I'm writing all of this. It seems ludicrous. I can't even begin to imagine what's going to happen.

Dear Journal,

Well, here I am. I'm alive. I think constantly about everything that's happening. This morning I was sitting at the front desk at work having panic attacks. I'd forget that I was pregnant for a little bit and then I'd suddenly remember. My heart would start pounding and I'd feel weak and shaky. Luckily we didn't have too many appointments and the waiting room was mostly empty. I was glad that I didn't have to concentrate on work very hard because this is all I can think about right now.

Mom called and said she got me an appointment for Friday morning with a doctor she used to go to. I had to call her last night and tell her, because I knew I needed to see a doctor and I don't have one. I didn't know how she'd react, but she was surprisingly calm and didn't freak out like I expected. I didn't want to say outright that I'm pregnant, so I told her that I haven't had a period in eight weeks and want to see a doctor. I'm sure she saw right through it. She just asked me in this low quiet voice if I thought I might be pregnant. What could I say? I've never lied to my parents. I told her I might be. I couldn't bring myself to tell her that I've already taken a home pregnancy test and know that I definitely am. After that all she said was that she guessed I didn't save myself for marriage. I felt about an inch high when I said yes. They have taught me all my life that sex is for marriage and premarital sex is sin. We've known that all along, and still we couldn't control ourselves. But even then she didn't say much. She said she would call a doctor and try to get me an appointment. The whole thing wasn't as bad as I thought it would be. But I know she's told Dad and for that reason I dread the weekend. I'll be going home Friday night and I have to face my family. Mom's going to come into the city and take me to the appointment. What a good mom.

I told my boss, Caroline, and some of the other girls at work overheard, so they know, too. Caroline is really understanding. I feel like I can talk to her openly about everything. The other girls seem fine with the news. No one has been judgmental, only interested in my well-being. I'm glad that the clinic is one place I can go to and feel completely safe. No one will think badly of me or look down on me there. What a relief, since I'll be spending most of my time there.

I talked to Phill for a long time again this evening. I called him last night and told him the test was positive. I don't think he was really surprised. He's terrified of telling his parents. He told his sister Elizabeth just because he had to tell somebody.

I'm pretty much feeling okay at the moment, but I don't think I know yet how bad things are going to get or how much will be wrecked or changed. Will we get married and raise our child? Or will we give it up for adoption and continue on? I am trying to trust God to guide us. It will be difficult, but it won't kill us. We will survive and our love will survive, and eventually things will get better. I really wonder what Dad is thinking. His reaction will be the hardest to predict and get through.

You know, I've never believed in abortion and I grew up being taught that it's wrong. But in the past day and a half, I suddenly realized why some girls think it's an attractive option. I can understand why they would want it all to be over so they wouldn't have to deal with all the things I'm dealing with right now. The thing is, I know it's never over after an abortion. That stuff haunts you for your whole life.

Dear Journal,

This weekend will be one of the worst of my life, if not *the* worst. Mom called again. She said that if the result is positive tomorrow at the doctor's appointment (and I already know it will be), then we are going to get together with Phill's parents on Sunday to talk to them about it. How will I survive that? I'll have to sit there and endure four opinions of me and what I should do instead of only my parents' two. And she also said, regardless of whether or not it's positive, she and Dad want to have a talk with me. That scares me for a few reasons. Are they going to figure out how long this has been going on? Or about the lies I told them and the innocence I pretended? I'm going to die. I'm going to ruin our relationship and I'll never be able to talk to them about anything again because I'll feel so guilty. They'll never trust me again. Every time Mom would question me about my physical relationship with Phill, I'd make it seem like she had nothing to be concerned about and that I was so innocent. But how could I have told her? I never would have felt comfortable enough to tell her the truth. I just always hoped that she'd never find out. And now she'll know. Everyone will know. My younger sister, Jo, is going to be so mad at me. What kind of example am I setting for her?

Are we going to be forced into doing something against our will? Will our parents pick a wedding date for us? What are we going to do? I know that we've ruined and changed so many things in so many people's lives. I can't even imagine the extent of it. Am I going to be miserable for the next year? Are Phill and I ever going to be able to see each other on weekends again? Will I have to raise a child when I feel like only a child myself?

For a few brief moments today, I fantasized about running away. I thought it would be easier to tell Phill to come pick me up in the middle of the night and just drive somewhere far away where no one else would have to deal with this except the two of us—the ones who deserve it—somewhere where we wouldn't have to hear what other people think of us. One of the hardest things about this whole situation, which I had never thought of before, is how hard this is for everyone around us. Our families and friends have to deal with this hardship almost as much as we do. I wish I could bear the weight of it all alone and spare those around me. I soon realized that running off alone isn't realistic and would make things much worse. We're going to need people to help us get through the next nine months.

Dear Journal,

Everything is getting harder and harder. Mom took me to my appointment today with Dr. Michiko. She said I'm already eight weeks pregnant. My due date is February 25. We went out for lunch, then I went back to work. Phill called me there to ask how it went, and all I could do was cry. Caroline told me to take the rest of the day off, so I went home and slept for three hours.

I dreaded going home to my parents' in the evening but it ended up not being so bad. When I walked in the door I was afraid to look at Dad's face, but he just came up to me and hugged me for a long time with tears in his eyes. He didn't say anything about it until we had "the talk" later. What he basically told me is that adoption is out, that we should get married and give this baby a wonderful home. It sounded so easy and perfect the way he said it.

But talking to Phill is getting worse. I cried the whole time. He isn't ready for marriage and a family at all. He feels all alone because everyone else thinks we should get married, including me. He's scared and feels like no one understands him. It also upsets him that my parents won't even let us consider adoption. I feel terrible for him. He asked me what I want, but the only thing I really know that I want is him and that everything will be okay between us. I hate how we differ in opinion. I agreed with what Dad said, but Phill doesn't want marriage and kids. It makes me wonder if I was fooling myself all along, thinking that he's the one I wanted to marry and have kids with, and now I find out he doesn't even want that. He's going to feel so bad on Sunday if he has to tell everyone that marriage is not what he wants. But he also said that he wants to make himself open to what God wants. If God wants us to get married, will He help change Phill's feelings about it? I've been crying so much. Can our baby handle all this stress? I need to pray.

Dear Journal,

Phill came over today and we went to the city. We went out for lunch and saw a stupid movie. He was being very lovable, hugging me and holding my hand. But the closer we got to home, the slower he drove. When we pulled up to the house, he said he'd had enough for one day and went home. When he called me at nine, he was very depressed and didn't say much. What am I supposed to do? I feel useless. I didn't know what to say.

Mom and Dad came and talked to me again. They said they thought about it and have changed their minds about adoption. It's our decision, and they'll respect what we decide. And we don't have to decide tomorrow when Phill's parents come over. But when I told Phill what they had said about changing their minds, he barely even responded. I wonder if I should call him back. Maybe he'll want to marry me when I'm eight-months pregnant, though I doubt it.

Dear Journal,

Today wasn't such a bad day. Phill's parents came down and, to my relief, we didn't have to participate in the discussion. So Phill and I watched TV in the basement and they talked for a long time upstairs. After supper they let us in on their conclusions. They said we'd all have to do a lot of praying, forgiving, and trusting God. Phill's dad suggested we get engaged, but said it was only a suggestion, whatever that means. It wasn't really clear to me what they want.

Phill wasn't so depressed today. We were able to talk and have fun. He took me back to the city on his motorcycle. He still doesn't think that he's ready for marriage, but somehow I think that, sometime down the road, he may change his mind. Dare I say it? In a way, I would like to get married and raise our little one, but if he just can't, then I'll live.

Dear Journal,

Phill and I talked on the phone until 1:30 last night. We were talking about adoption. By the end, I was bawling and he felt so rotten. He thinks it's what we should do, whereas I was hysterical just thinking about it. He felt so bad that he began to put himself down, saying that I need someone better who would love this baby. It got to the point where he said he doesn't think our relationship will make it, because we see things so differently. He thinks I want to get married and keep the baby. But I don't think he quite understands how I'm really thinking, and I couldn't find the words to explain myself to him. Yes, I would probably prefer to marry and keep our baby, but I don't know if that's right or the best thing to do. And in that, I'm willing to change my mind so that everything works out for us. I have seven months to get used to the idea of adoption, and we would choose a loving Christian home for our child. But he said that the bigger the baby gets, the more I'll be attached to it and the less we'll agree. I'm not sure that'll be the case. Of course it will be hard and I'll need him so much, but the important thing to me is to not let this drive us apart. At all costs, I hope that we will love each other, maybe even more, in the end.

Dear Journal,

Last night when Phill and I talked, he mentioned a couple that he knows of who are looking to adopt a baby. These people are good friends of his oldest sister, Marianne. He even asked Marianne about them, and she said they'd be very excited to take our baby. She said they are excellent people. It makes us both feel better. I hope we're headed in the right direction, and I hope our parents will support us. I still have a lot of mixed feelings about adoption. I'm not totally convinced that this is the right thing to do or that this is what God wants us to do, but it doesn't hurt to explore options, right?

Dear Journal,

On Sunday, Phill and I went to see the pastor of my church and his wife, who are my Uncle Henry and Aunt Kate. They wanted to have a talk with us, so we went over to their house after lunch. I was dreading it because I knew what they would probably say. It was not very comfortable. While I just sat there in quiet distress, Phill defended himself and his reasoning, and the whole conversation seemed to be getting nowhere. They really seemed to push marriage without actually coming right out and saying it. Phill was very discouraged when we left. It's really making me have more doubts about adoption. And now, here's a new dilemma: how do I face my own pastor knowing that he thinks my decision is wrong? There's no way I could confide in him now, or ask his advice, or anything. Besides that, they are my relatives, whom I've known all my life and have always been comfortable with. Now we have this between us, and it makes everything very awkward.

August

Dear Journal,

It's been a stressful Saturday evening. Mom and Dad gave me another talk; this time they were worried about my relationship with Phill. They were concerned that he went home at 6:30 today instead of his usual late departure. I hadn't thought anything of it and tried to reassure them that it wasn't a big deal.

I think our biggest problem is our relationship with God. I need to get serious about reading my Bible and praying continuously. I spend a lot of time at the piano nowadays, playing hymns and choruses and singing. Playing piano has always been kind of a therapy for me; it helps me think through things. Lately I've really been paying attention to the words the composers have written in their hymns. They seem to have so much faith, letting God bend them in any direction. I want to be like that, even if I'm scared of what that might mean.

My other concern is Phill—he is praying, isn't he? Does he read his Bible? When was the last time he was in church? How then, if he doesn't do any of these things, does he expect to make a sure decision? Sometimes I feel like everything rests on him. If he would just say the word, we'd get married and everything would turn out happily ever after. I'm praying for God to soften his heart and make him vulnerable to His will, but what part can I play? I feel like our entire lives are subject to what we end up deciding. If I get serious about praying, what can God do? Can I trust Him enough?

Dear Journal,

Why can't anyone leave me alone? Why must people gossip and speculate? Why can't they keep their opinions to themselves? Why do they have to know everything? I've only known for three weeks! Why do they do all these things and then say they're trying to encourage me? How much does Phill love me? How much faith does he have? Where is my miracle? When will God rescue me? Why didn't I run away? Why doesn't anyone answer any of my questions? Will Phill ask me to marry him? How much does he pray? Does he pray for me? Why can't he do it? Why do I want to so much? What will be the end of all this? Why do I feel alone and trapped? Why do I still feel guilty? Where is God? What is He saying to me? Is He saying anything? Why don't I know? Why didn't I know any better?

Dear Journal,

I had a long talk with Phill about our situation. I don't think we realize just how hard these next months will be and just how many things we may ruin. So far, adoption is still the best choice. It's the only way I see things working out. Sometimes I feel like I'm going to bawl and lose control when I think about it, but other times I feel so confident.

My co-workers seem to be in worse situations than me: one's mother passed away last night; another wants to leave her husband but is afraid he will be violent; another just left her husband and might be getting a divorce. So I suppose being pregnant and giving my baby to excellent people isn't so bad.

There's something else that bugs me. A few people have asked me, "Why didn't you use birth control?" First, I can't believe these people had the nerve to even ask me that. Second, I didn't want to use birth control. I knew that what we were doing was just plain wrong and I thought that birth control would be sort of the "ticket to ride." We were trying to stop having sex, not just cover it up with birth control so we wouldn't get caught. For some reason, they just can't understand that.

Dear Journal,

This evening Uncle Henry and Aunt Kate came over to my apartment to talk to me again. I find it funny how this time they didn't want to talk to Phill too. Ever since our last talk, I can't help but try to avoid them in church. I love them as my aunt and uncle, but I can't stand the awkwardness of the situation, and I'm always so afraid they'll want to talk about it some more. I guess they figure if they come to my apartment I can't say no or run away from them! This time it wasn't so bad; it was actually somewhat encouraging, but I still just feel nervous and weird around them. They wanted to talk about this coming Sunday. Dad really encouraged me from the beginning to go up in church and tell everyone what's going on. He said I need to ask for forgiveness from my church family and clear up any speculation. I agree with him... mostly about the speculation part. I've heard from my mom how gossipy my church can be, and I know there are a select few who would run away with information like this. It's actually really sad that I can't even depend on my church family for unconditional support. Church is the first place I should be able to go for help, and here I am planning to tell them all that I'm pregnant, just so they won't gossip about me.

So that's happening this Sunday, and I guess Uncle Henry just wanted to make sure I knew what to say and stuff like that. But every time I talk to them, I'm reminded how difficult this situation is. I need a miracle!

Dear Journal,

This morning in church, at the end of the service, I went up to the front and said my thing about being pregnant and wanting forgiveness. I went through every emotion possible while I sat waiting for the end of the service: fear, nervousness, sadness, even excitement. But I was able to do it. I had almost expected there to be a big unanimous gasp when Uncle Henry told everyone that I was pregnant, but I didn't hear a sound. When I went up to speak I could hardly see what I was reading because of the tears in my eyes, but I managed. I kept it short and simple. All I told them was that I am pregnant, I know the circumstances that brought me to the present situation are wrong, and I need forgiveness. I ended with 1 Corinthians 15:57: *"But thanks be to God, which giveth us the victory through our Lord Jesus Christ."* Many people were crying when I sat down.

I was so glad Phill decided to come. He's been afraid of coming to my church because of what people have been saying about him, and I don't blame him. I think a lot of my older male cousins felt really protective of me when they heard I was pregnant, and naturally they would blame Phill and think badly of him. He's never felt comfortable with them to begin with, and he hasn't been coming to my church as often as he used to. I guess they concluded that he'd abandoned me or something. It's just not fair that they don't bother to ask and find out the truth. But despite all of this, Phill was there today, holding my hand and whispering in my ear. And a lot of people came up to us after the service with hugs and encouragement.

In the evening, once I was back at my apartment in the city, Phill called me. Sometimes he gets me down because I wonder if he's as devoted to me as I am to him. I don't think that he likes to go out with me as much any more; he says it feels different and it's not as good a time any more. That really scares me. I still believe most times that marriage and keeping the baby is really the answer, but then I put myself in his position and I can see why he doesn't want anything to do with it. I feel really lost, and I don't know what will happen. In the end, will we even still be together?

Dear Journal,

I thought yesterday would be the last day of my life, but as it turns out, I'm still alive. I told Phill how I feel about adoption and how I would like to get married instead. It was so terrible. I feel worse than I've ever felt in my whole life for the position it puts us in. I almost thought it would be the end of us. I cried and cried until one o'clock in the morning. How will we ever stay together if we can't agree on this? It's like a huge brick wall that stands between us. There's no such thing as a compromise in this situation; it's either one or the other.

I've been nervous all day about phoning him again. It was my day off today, so I did some shopping and went out for supper with Teresa and Karen. By the time we got back, Phill had already tried to call me twice. When I called him back, he seemed fairly cheerful. We didn't talk about last night. It's easier to talk about other things besides the baby than to rip ourselves apart trying to figure the situation out. In some ways, it's very relieving to just set it aside and think about something else for awhile.

Dear Journal,

I think Phill and I are doing okay now. We didn't talk about anything today concerning adoption or the baby. We still don't know what to do. Something I've noticed about Phill is the more someone tries to convince him of something, the less and less he is willing to listen or be convinced. No one can force him to do or decide anything. He ends up resenting whoever is trying to change his mind. I'm just going to have to let him figure things out for himself. I have to wait and trust God. He is the only one who can help Phill turn around, if that's what's right. Everything is so confusing.

Dear Journal,

I need to call Phill yet tonight. It seems every night when I talk to him and we discuss our situation, I end up crying and he ends up feeling rotten. He's losing hope. What are we going to do? It seems like adoption is the only solution that will solve anything. Maybe it's the only way Phill and I can stay together.

Tomorrow I have another doctor's appointment. I'm mostly scared that hearing the baby's heartbeat will make me really want to keep it and it'll make everything worse. All I can think when I think about adoption is how much I love Phill and want us to be happy together.

Dear Journal,

This morning was my appointment. It was quick and painless. I heard the baby's heartbeat. Boy, that little guy's just going in there! Even though I feared hearing the heartbeat, it didn't affect me like I thought it would. Dr. Michiko measured him too, but she never said how big he is. She's getting me an ultrasound appointment, but who knows when that will be. I also had blood taken again. They have to do that every visit because I'm Rh-negative.

Dear Journal,

The doctor's office called me this morning. My ultrasound is September 18 at 4:45 p.m. Not as late as I thought it would be. I've thought a little bit about names. I think, with open adoption, we would get to choose the second name. I'm thinking of Russell for a boy and Colby or Bianca for a girl.

Questions for Phill:

- Does this situation in any way make you want to spend less time with me? If so, what is the reason for it?
- Are we going to be able to deal with our decision?
- Is our love going to get stronger or weaker by the end?
- Are you going to be there when I need you, with no hesitation?
- Are we going to be able to handle the things that change and the ways we change?
- Are we always going to be on the same side?

Positive ways to look at this pregnancy:

- If someone re-evaluates their physical relationship by what I've been going through, it's worth it.
- If Phill and I grow up and grow stronger, it's worth it.
- If our physical stuff slows down and our spiritual life gets better, it's worth it.
- If we make someone happy and help answer their prayers, it's worth it.

Dear Journal,

I had the day off and went with Jo and my parents to move her into the residence at her high school. It's the same school Phill and I graduated from, and I talked to a lot of my old teachers. Every time someone asked me if I was still dating Phill, I thought, "Uh, yeah, actually I'm three-and-a-half-months pregnant with his child!" I wondered what their reaction would be if I told them. Mostly I just hoped no one would notice that my waistline isn't as small as it once was.

I don't fit in any of my pants anymore. Jo and Mom gave me some of their clothes, but I think I'll have to buy some stretchy pants.

September

Dear Journal,

I'm worried about Phill. He has a lot of sad and frustrating days. He tells me that we've not only changed the present and future but the past, as well. Everything is depressing for him. His aunts, uncles, and cousins don't know that I'm pregnant yet, so he doesn't even want me to come over any more, in case someone would see me and find out—even though I'm hardly showing yet. I just wish there was something I could do to make him happy.

Lately I've been thinking about my dreams and what I want to accomplish in my lifetime. I think someday I might want to go to university, buy a car, or build my dream country farmhouse. But the more realistically I think about it, the more I just want Phill and me to be happy. If adoption is what it takes for this to happen, then maybe that's what we should do.

Then I think of what I read in my devotions the other night and wonder, would God put us through this if He didn't want to refine us, make us stronger and more devoted to him? The devotion said trials in life are designed to refine us and purify us like gold by the time we come out the other side.[1]

Dear Journal,

Phill called me this evening from his parents' farm. He was combining canola at the time, and I think he's got a lot of thinking time when he's sitting out there on the field on the combine. I think he's had second thoughts about adoption. He couldn't explain to me exactly how he felt, but he mentioned something about his cousin and his son. I don't think we will have a final decision until the baby's born.

Dear Journal,

Ever since Phill made that comment to me about his cousin's little boy that made me think he's having second thoughts, I've really been thinking: if we decide to keep our baby, am I prepared to suddenly deal with that? The last few weeks, all I've been thinking about is adoption, and I'm getting really used to the idea. Deciding to keep the baby opens up a whole new set of questions and problems that we haven't discussed so far. Where would we live? How would we make money? Would we be married? Or would I be taking care of the baby on my own? I know nothing about babies or how to take care of them.

Dear Journal,

One thing that has been bothering me today is that people, namely Jo and Jodi, keep dropping hints that they expect me to keep my baby. I'm home for the weekend and my parents' neighbour Jodi was over. They talk about things, just assuming that we're going to keep it. Then Jo and I went for a walk and, for some reason, we were talking about baby strollers. I made a comment, something about not needing a stroller for a long time, and she just looked at me and said, "Yes, you will." She said it rather forcefully and really took me by surprise. It makes me angry to think that she wouldn't be understanding enough to let us make our own decision, especially not knowing every aspect of the situation we're in.

I'm beginning to be afraid of everyone. How will I go to Jo's Christmas concert with all my old teachers there? Teresa invited me to the youth group she goes to, but there are a lot of people there I used to know. Everyone will notice that I'm pregnant. What would they think of me then? How would Phill feel, telling people about his girlfriend who is massive, moody, and eats like a pig? I'm going to be so embarrassed of myself.

Another thing I'm afraid of is maternity clothes! They are all hideous, and I am never going to find anything to wear that makes me look, or feel, even half decent. But the worst thing of all that I have to endure is other people's opinions! This may be what kills me.

Dear Journal,

Today was the ultrasound. Phill took me to the appointment. When we got to the hospital, I had to put on a gown and lie on a bed. Phill wasn't allowed to come in with me at that point. The nurse put a bunch of goo on my belly and took forty pictures of the baby for the program on the computer. After that was all over, Phill came in and we got to see our baby moving. He yawned and stretched and rubbed his head. The cutest part was when he scratched his nose. He weighs eight ounces and is ten centimetres long. She printed some pictures of his face and feet for me. In one picture he is yawning. I never did find out what the gender is, but I assume it's a boy. I don't know; I just have this feeling.

I can't go anywhere or do anything without thinking about the difficulty we're facing. Even during the ultrasound, the nurse referred to Phill as my husband by accident and gave me all sorts of child-care advice. I didn't have the heart to tell her that we aren't married and we don't think we're going to keep the baby. Why bother? People in general just assume that everything's fine, that we're a happy family having our first child. It's frustrating for me to listen to people who don't know me ask if I've finished the baby's nursery or if I'm excited. What am I supposed to say? "No, I'm not excited"? I usually don't bother telling them the truth. I just go along with whatever they say. But every time it happens my insides churn and I wish they had never said anything.

After the ultrasound, we went out for supper and came back to my apartment to dye Phill's hair. He left at 8:00. He just started university this week, and he's living with his friend Tim until they have possession of their apartment. So he called me later for help with one of his assignments. It really scares me to think of January when he'll be stressed about school and we'll have to decide what to do with the baby. In some ways I think, how could we give it up? This is a special life created by God and given to us as a blessing. It's a part of both of us, meant for both of us. But on the other hand, when things get rough, it just comes down to the fact that I love Phill and we have to stay together.

Dear Journal,

I'm definitely suffering from pregnancy insanity. I get irritated very easily. The clients at work are very frustrating sometimes. I finally got off work at 7:30 this evening, then I went to get a few groceries. Once home, I felt so worn out. I have a cold, but I can't take anything for it. I don't even know if cough drops are safe! And Karen's boyfriend is here and they're cuddling on the couch. I don't want to disturb them, but I don't want to be stuck in this bedroom all evening! To top off my bad day, I called

Phill's cellphone only to discover that he is playing Nintendo at his friend's place and can't talk to me. I really wanted to have a real conversation with him today. Lately he's been so busy with homework that I feel like we haven't really had a good talk in a long time. I'm afraid that this is what it will turn out to be: the nearer I get to my due date, the less we'll talk, the busier he'll be, and the less he'll want to deal with a pregnant girlfriend and a decision about a baby. And yet, for all the hurdles in our relationship that I saw coming in the past, not one has knocked us down yet.

Dear Journal,

I feel disturbed. I went to my cousin's place today and we talked a lot about pregnancy and childbirth, since she has a six-month-old boy. The things she said about birth scare me. I feel like I don't know anything. The thought of giving birth completely terrifies me, and the more I'm around babies and think about babies, the less I want one. I feel guilty for that, but I can't help it. Sometimes I even have this horrible thought that I'll be somewhat relieved to give the baby to someone else. I can't believe I actually wrote that; it seems so wrong. Poor Phill is so busy with school, he's sick, plus he has everything else to worry about.

I had another doctor's appointment. It went fine. I should find out about prenatal classes at the hospital. But I need a partner, or a "coach," and I don't know who to ask. I don't think Phill wants to do it. The thought of birth scares him more than it scares me. If not Phill, the only person I can think of is Karen.

Dear Journal,

Last night when I was lying in bed I felt the baby move for the first time. I was on my back staring at the ceiling and thinking, with my hand on my stomach. And then under my hand I felt this tiny little poke, like a little foot or hand was pressing upward. It was so small that I almost didn't feel it. Half of me was thrilled, and the other half was sad. If the circumstances were different, I could really be excited about it, but as it is now, I'm almost afraid to be.

October

Dear Journal,

I helped Phill and Tim move into their apartment the other day. I was always so excited that Phill would be moving into the city, because I thought we'd get to see each other more. But the way he's been busy lately, that may not happen.

One thing that bugs me about our situation is that I want my life to be changed when it's all over. If we give up the baby and I just go back to working full-time, I'll feel like nothing's changed and it had no purpose. I guess I'm expecting that God has something big to teach us through all of this. If I just go back to work and put it behind me after the baby's born, I'll feel like I didn't learn a thing.

Dear Journal,

I'm really looking forward to our family's big Thanksgiving gathering. I'm hoping to talk to my cousin Lauren if she's there. She gave up her first baby for adoption a few years ago, and I have so many questions for her. Why did she give up her baby? How did she feel about it later? How long did it take her to get back into things? Would she recommend adoption to me?

A nurse from the hospital returned my call about prenatal classes. I think I'll call Jodi and ask her to be my coach. We've been friends for a long time, even though she's older, and she's had three kids, so at least she knows what to expect.

Phill won't answer his phone and I really want to talk to him. My kid has been going crazy the past few days. I can feel him poking and nudging all the time. Sometimes it feels like bubbles popping in my stomach.

Dear Journal,

Before my brother James picked me up to go home for the weekend, I called Phill. He kept going on and on about this girl he knows, Sara, and her friends who live below him and Tim, and how they went to the bar last night and how he had to shut down this girl who asked him to dance the last song.... The way he talked made me glad that he's happy and having fun but sort of depressed about myself. He's so lucky that he can get away from his problems and live a different life, while I'm stuck with this pregnancy 24/7 and I can't ever get away from it. What fun is it turning down pretty girls at a bar and remembering that you have a pregnant girlfriend you're stuck with? He even admitted that it's like he lives two lives; one life is fun and carefree, and the other is me—moody me, someone who reminds him of his problems every time he looks at her. At times I wish so badly that I could have a fun life that I could live, like he has. But what do I have? I don't have friends that I go out with. I couldn't go to a bar even if I wanted to. I feel like the more pregnant I get, the more detached I'll become from a social life and maybe even from Phill. Why would he want to be around me if I just remind him of his problems and drag him down? I want him to be happy. But I want to be happy too, and I'm not sure how long it'll be before I actually will be happy. I keep thinking about our baby, and how he or she will one day respond to the decision that we're making, and how I'll think of him every day.

Dear Journal,

Every time I come home for the weekend, I just hope against hope that Mom and Dad won't want to have another "talk." I guess deep down I knew they wouldn't keep quiet forever. After supper today, they finally said what they've been thinking. They think that our decision to give the baby up for adoption is really just Phill's decision and I'm giving everything up just to make him happy. They said a lot more, but that was basically the point. I cried and cried. Then Phill called me at the end and we talked about it all. I asked why, exactly, he didn't want the baby. The more he said, the more Mom and Dad made sense. He sounded very self-centered. When I told him that "I just can't" isn't a reason, he said that he didn't want to talk any more, so we hung up. We were both very upset.

Now I really wonder if he'll ever want to phone me or see me again. The ironic thing is that I actually felt better after we hung up. I felt that, for the first time, I was completely honest with him and did something right, like I took a step in the right direction. I keep waiting for the guilt to come, the regret that I've upset him and perhaps jeopardized us, but it hasn't come yet. The truth is that I don't think I have wrecked everything by what I said. But I do know that my crying isn't over and the hardship has only begun. Phill may never agree with me. I also feel very sorry about the position he's in. No one agrees with him; he has no one to talk to, and people will blame him and look down on him for this. I've already made up my mind to defend him if need be. From now on, my life may drastically change.

Dear Journal,

I've been so depressed and miserable all day. All I can think about is Phill and how much I miss him. It was crushing, sitting at home all afternoon with him not there and no hope of possibly seeing him today or tomorrow. I feel useless and meaningless, and I've been close to tears all day. Finally I told Mom that I wanted to go back to the city to my apartment, so she and Dad drove me in, even though I have tomorrow off. I don't even have any idea what I'll do here all day tomorrow by myself. Maybe it's just the thought that I'm a little closer to Phill, since I know he's still here at his apartment. I don't know if I should call him or if I should just wait until he calls me.

This whole situation remains unsolved. I don't know what to do. I keep begging God to give me an answer, but I can't seem to hear any response. Maybe I'm not listening hard enough. The idea of adoption just doesn't seem right, but keeping the baby seems impossible. When I think about a baby and all that taking care of one involves, sometimes I want nothing to do with one. Even the thought of living at home with my parents for the first while after he's born seems very unappealing. But I still can't shake the feeling or the idea that that's what I should do. And where does that leave Phill? Even if we didn't marry right away, he'd feel a lot of pressure that we had to. What if he never wants to? I guess that would mean that he isn't the one for me, which will destroy me. Mom said that maybe this is all a test for Phill.

But he's going to feel like I'm against him, when before I was the only one who stood with him. He'll think no one understands him, and he'll hate my parents and think they turned me against him. Everyone will look down on him for not supporting what I think is right, and he'll be a wreck. If only I could spare him. I don't want him to think that he's not as important to me as a baby, but I can't live with making a decision I think is wrong. Sometimes thinking about it is so discouraging that I want to just give in to him again. But I can't now. Am I going to end up losing him? Would I anyway, even if I did give in? Dad said the worst thing I can do to myself is try to do everything Phill's way just to try to make him happy. But what else is there to do that won't end in a lifetime of agony? I can't even begin to come up with a solution to this problem. I don't want to place the baby for adoption, but I'm way too scared to say that I'm going to keep him for sure. Nothing will ever be the same again, no matter what we do. Why don't we pick the option that everyone will support? How does Phill know he would never love this child or be a good father? And why is it that a baby will make him stop loving me?

Dear Journal,

I ended up calling Phill last night, and our conversation was fairly normal. I spent all day at his place today. We didn't really talk about the situation very much, but he did say a couple of things. He made it very clear that he does not want to get married right now. He also said he hopes I don't keep the baby, because if I do, he'll feel pressured that we'd have to get married. That sounded pretty selfish to me. But if I keep the baby, there's no way we'd have to get married right away.

Mom called after Phill dropped me off, and she was pretty insistent that I tell Phill very soon that I'm keeping the baby no matter what. I'm reluctant, though. I hate to do that to him. I feel awful already about hurting him. I don't know what to do. God help us.

Dear Journal,

I'm terrified about telling Phill that I'm keeping the baby. Every time I think about it, I get panicky. One thing I know is that I don't want to tell him on the phone. I'd rather tell him in person, even if he gets really upset and tells me to leave or something like that. At least I could cry all the way home on the bus instead of sitting through a ten-minute telephone silence. He's going to have a fit; I know he will. How, then, will I tell him all the things I need to tell him, if he's yelling at me? Would he yell at me? I don't even know. All I know is that he's going to be very upset. But I want to tell him that I love him, and I'm terribly sorry for the position it puts him in, and I don't expect a wedding ring—that's entirely up to him. He may hate me forever and never want to see me again, but I know it's the right thing to do and I won't ever regret keeping my baby. I desperately hope that Phill won't be heartbroken and hate me, but I know it's a possibility, and I have to be realistic. I don't know what I'd do without him. But maybe I'm jumping to conclusions here. I actually don't know what he'll do or say, and I shouldn't just write him off before I hear it.

Dear Journal,

Last night, in the middle of my writing, Phill called. We had a horrible argument. I didn't have to announce that I was keeping the baby. He already knew that it was on my mind. We argued for an hour. I cried the whole time, and I bawled for a whole hour after we hung up. I seriously don't think I can do what Mom and Dad want me to. To say to him that I'm keeping the baby regardless of what he thinks is the same as telling him that I don't love him and don't care about his feelings. It's the same as throwing our whole three years away. If I love him so much, I just can't do that. But how can I give up our baby? This dilemma has plagued me ever since we talked, and I cannot for the life of me come up with any solution.

At the end of our conversation last night, we agreed to take a week apart from each other and see how we feel in the end. No seeing each other; no phone calls; nothing. Before we hung up, he said how much he loves me, how he'll miss me and think about me. He said it so sweetly and tenderly. It hurts unbelievably to argue like this.

This situation is absolutely impossible! I can't lose him! I just can't! No matter what I do, I'm going to end up losing or hurting someone, whether it'll be Phill, the baby, or my parents. I'm most afraid of talking to them. I always clam up when they sit me down. I won't be able to defend our case; I'll just sit there and cry. I'm scared to call Mom, because then I'll have to tell her that I haven't done what they want me to do.

I'm not sure if it was stress or what, but when I got to work this morning, I felt awful. My stomach hurt so bad, the pain was shooting into my legs and hips and I felt dizzy and nauseous. So I made an emergency trip to the doctor, who told me that I'm fine—I'm just pregnant. My blood pressure is practically non-existent, and she thought my hemoglobin had dropped. The stomach pain is my uterus stretching. She also said that my baby is above-average size for its age and will probably end up being eight pounds. I can't deliver an eight-pound kid!

Now I have to wait a week before talking to or seeing Phill. It seems like an eternity. But in the meantime, I plan on doing some research. I talked to one of the vets at work today, and she said that adoption is the most selfless thing I could do. She assured me that it's a good idea and not wrong at all. But she also believes in evolution, so I don't know how seriously I should take her advice. I also plan on going to the Pregnancy Crisis Centre on Monday and hopefully will get enough courage to call my cousin Lauren.

The worst thing about adoption is telling Mom and Dad. But the alternative is much worse: losing Phill. Like I said, no matter what path I choose, I end up hurting someone.

Dear Journal,

I've had sort of a tough evening. I wrote letters to both Phill and my parents, explaining to each of them how I'm feeling. I told Phill in his letter that I love him and can't throw our relationship away. I can't disregard his opinion in this decision. In my parents' letter, I apologized and told them the same thing. I'm so scared to see or talk to my parents. I feel pressured by them, and I'm scared of doing the opposite of what they want. I was hoping to take the bus down to Phill's apartment while he's at school and put his letter under a windshield wiper on his car, but I'd probably set off the alarm. I miss him a lot. He's all I can think of. I can't wait to see him next week. Now I'm scared of going home. I'm not sure if I can talk to my parents.

Dear Journal,

I love my dear journal. No matter what time of day, no matter what's happening, it's always waiting for me to pick it up and complain to it or cry to it or rejoice to it. Besides Phill, it's my best friend. It will never give me an opinion but it will listen to anything and everything I have to say.

Work was very slow. One of Phill's friends took Teresa out in the evening. I asked if he had talked to Phill lately but he said no. Phill's toughest exam was today. I miss him a lot. When I see him again, I'm going to tell him that I love him and ask him to please forgive me for all the awful things I said. I can't wait until I can put my arms around him again.

All this evening I've been bothered by intense lower back and side pain. At times it has me in tears. The baby must be hitting a nerve.

I went home this evening. I feel like I've been walking on thin ice; at any moment, my parents will want to say something to me or have another big "talk." But much to my relief, they haven't said anything. I would like to be left alone for awhile. Forever, actually, but I know they can't wait that long.

Dear Journal,

One of my cousins got engaged today. It was really romantic. He got his friend to take them up in an airplane; then they flew over a field where a bunch of bales were set up to spell out "Marry me." Right when they flew over, James and some other people lit the bales on fire.

We were at my aunt's place at the time, and the happy couple showed up, beaming and showing off the ring. I thought all the marriage excitement would make me very sad in view of my situation, but it really didn't. Then I thought maybe Mom and Dad would be thinking the same thing, but I tried to ignore those thoughts.

This back pain won't go away. I'm only five-and-a-half-months pregnant and my belly feels stretched to the limit. How am I going to deal with a nine-months-pregnant body? I really miss Phill and am growing more convinced that I need to stand by his side no matter what. When I see him this week, I'm going to give him a big hug and tell him I love him.

Dear Journal,

It's Sunday morning and my family is at church without me. My back hurt so much last night that I barely slept more than half an hour all night. The wheat bag is the only thing giving me some relief.

I'm beginning to understand where Phill's opinions are coming from. We have been looking at this situation from two completely different angles; his view is logical and mine is emotional. All of my arguments have been based on a feeling, but if I think logically about everything Phill's said, I can understand what he's saying and why he's said it. It's not that he doesn't care about me or the baby. It's just that he's really and honestly figuring out in his head what can and can't be done and what is best.

I put the letter I wrote to my parents on my bed when I left to go back to the city. I'm nervous about it, but what can I do?

Dear Journal,

Jodi came into the city today and took me shopping. Before she dropped me off, we sat in her car and had a big talk about my situation. I don't mind it so much, coming from her, but everything is so complicated and now she's given me even more to think about. This seems to be my choice: do I keep this baby and risk leaving Phill behind? Or do I have enough faith in our love that I can confidently give the baby up? I really want to see him tomorrow.

Dear Journal,

Before I went to work this morning, I took a bus downtown to the Pregnancy Crisis Centre. It is a really cozy place, very comfortable, so I didn't feel nervous at all. I talked to a lady named Lucy and she gave me a whole bunch of literature to read. I was telling her about the problems I've been having with my church family, and she thinks that Phill and I should find a church to go to together here in the city, where we can start fresh, in a sense. She also said we can come down and see her any time, and she'll even go with us to an adoption agency if we want her to.

Dear Journal,

I've finally talked to Phill! He called me at 9:30, and it's been so wonderful just to hear his voice. This past week has been the longest of my life. He's doing well on his exams, and he's done lots of thinking this week. I'm so proud of how honest, smart, and logical he's being. He told me that he needs me desperately, and I read him the letter I wrote him last week. I didn't know what he'd say, but he said he loved it. I missed him so much. I can't wait to see him. He said he was really nervous to talk to me today because he didn't want to make things worse.

Dear Journal,

I had a bad dream last night that I'm not going to forget about easily. I dreamt that I had our baby and kept it and then Phill sort of began to distance himself from me. He was at the bar with his friends all the time and wouldn't give me the time of day. It hurt me so badly. But now I keep thinking, how far from the truth could that scenario turn out to be? And what if we give it up? For how many weeks am I going to be depressed in my apartment, wanting to see Phill, and he'll tell me he's too busy with homework or has made plans with the guys? Sometimes I wonder if I will end up resenting him after all. I don't want to. But I'm stuck wondering how this experience will change our lives, our relationship, and about how I'm going to look back on this. Hindsight is 20/20, they say. Am I going to see something painfully obvious?

Dear Journal,

Phill called, but he sounded quite sad and we both had nothing to say. So it was a five-minute phone call. I really hope that after the baby comes I'll be understanding of his need for time to do homework and go out with his friends, but also that he'll want to be there for me. I wish I could sit down and talk to him about everything, but it seems like he's so busy with school that I can't even ask him to go out for coffee, just to talk with me. I don't know what's going to happen. I know there are many rough times ahead. But sometimes I read back over what I've written in this journal and think it sounds like I have no faith in Phill. I guess I just don't know how things will turn out. I have to believe that Phill loves me and needs me and that God is working His purposes out.

Dear Journal,

I'm pretty disappointed with this weekend. James came home to Mom and Dad's for lunch today, and then he drove me back to the city. I called Phill right away when I got to my apartment, in the hope that we could get together this afternoon. But he was in a bad mood and was rushing home to start on his homework. So that pretty much crushed all my hopes. I'm trying so hard to understand that he was upset and has lots of work to do and that I'd only distract him if I was there. I know it's not his fault that he has so much work to do. But I can't help but be very disappointed. I feel like we see each other less and less, and I wonder where that's going to put our situation and our relationship. Sometimes when I look at other people's relationships, I wonder if Phill and I will ever be normal or ever get married. Most of the time I feel like we don't quite get along lately; someone's always hurt or upset. I don't know whose fault that is. Should I be changing, or should he?

My parents never said anything about the letter I left them last weekend. But I know they must have read it, because it wasn't sitting on the bed where I left it. I hope it helped them understand, even just a little.

Dear Journal,

I called Phill's sister Marianne. She had a baby a few weeks ago and I wanted to see how she was doing. And I needed some encouragement. We talked for almost an hour. I feel like I can talk to her about anything, and she makes me feel so comfortable. She reassures me about things I am unsure about and gives me confidence. She is one of the few people in my life that I can turn to for real support and not worry about her judging me. When she found out I was pregnant, she went to the Pregnancy Crisis Centre near where she lives and picked up a whole package of information for Phill. She doesn't ask about what we're deciding; she just wants to know how I'm feeling. I really need that right now. I wish more people were like her.

I asked her about her friends David and Beth who are looking to adopt a baby. She told me everything she knew about open adoption and that they're registered with an agency here in the city. I was very glad to hear it. I think we need to go there and talk to someone about how it all works. But first I'd really like to talk to Phill and see what he thinks about everything. I hope he has time for that this week.

Take therefore no thought for the morrow: for the morrow shall take thought for the things of itself. (Matthew 6:34).

Dear Journal,

Phill ended up calling me at 9:30. He was still feeling bad, but he was okay to talk to. I'm going to his place tomorrow to help him study. He seemed excited about it. I also mentioned a few of the things Marianne told me. He thought that seeing David and Beth at the agency would be awkward since he's met them before, but I think he thought that going to the agency was a good idea. I think it's going to be hard, but I'm also really looking forward to it, maybe because it will seem like we're moving ahead.

My roommate Teresa gave me a book she got from her sister-in-law about how a baby grows in the womb, with tons of real-life colour photos. Right now my baby has hair, nails, wrinkly skin, and he can hear and respond to loud noises. I should soon be able to hear his heartbeat with a stethoscope and distinguish body parts when he moves. I'm twenty-four weeks now; that's about six months along.

Dear Journal,

I would really like to sit down with Phill and have a big serious talk about everything. I need to connect with him, since it seems like we haven't really *talked* in a long time. I'd also like for us to go to the adoption agency, maybe with Lucy from the Pregnancy Crisis Centre. But he's always so busy and he has so much homework. I feel like I'm adding pressure to his life, but this *has* to be dealt with. How on earth will it be, in February? What if he has to leave class because I'm in labour? Hello! Listen to me. That's a good enough reason to leave class! I'm just worried about the future.

November

Dear Journal,

I was halfway through my supper dishes when the doorbell rang, and there was Phill. He wanted me to help him study, but it turned out that he had brought the wrong books. Feeling quite stressed and frustrated, he stayed long enough to give me a hug and a kiss; then he went back home again. The poor boy, he has so much work to do and no time for anything else. I think he's feeling completely overwhelmed by his school work. I'm missing him a lot. It feels like we haven't really had a good conversation in ages.

Dear Journal,

I'm having sort of a sad evening. Today at work I picked up a magazine and stumbled on a story about a fourteen-year-old girl who got pregnant and kept her baby. Sure, she went through despair while her friends were going out and she had to stay at home and take care of a baby, but five years later she said it was the best thing she'd ever done. It makes me wonder, how is it that she kept her baby and I'm not keeping mine? If anyone would have a reason to give up a baby for adoption, it would be a fourteen year old whose boyfriend leaves and who still has to finish high school. If she did it, then why can't I? Am I totally blind and stupid?

Then when I got home and talked to Karen about it, she told me a story about a girl she knew who was determined to give her baby up for adoption. A week after he was born she went and took him back because she wanted him so badly. How am I going to feel after I give my baby away? What if Phill is so busy that he can't spend time with me and I have to deal with it alone? I'm terrified about what the future holds.

If I talk to my parents, they'll just encourage me to keep the baby and forget about Phill. So I guess I'm basically giving up the baby to save him and our relationship. Is that a bad reason? Although it's not as if I feel very strongly about keeping it, either. I'm so afraid of making a decision I'll regret the rest of my life. It would ruin me. Will adoption ruin me? I don't know the answers to any of these questions, and I won't know until I've already made a decision, right or wrong. When I think logically, my mind seems to lean toward adoption, but what if there is a big monster hiding behind those words, waiting to eat me?

For which cause we faint not; but though our outward man perish, yet the inward man is renewed day by day. (2 Corinthians 4:16).

Dear Journal,

I didn't feel like writing last night. The first prenatal class put me in a bad mood. It was really nice to have Jodi there, because she kept the atmosphere light with jokes and she kept making me laugh. Otherwise, I would have been utterly terrified. On the tour of the maternity ward, I felt awful. I felt like I was touring a prison I'd been sentenced to. The whole time, I thought, "This is where I'm going to be bawling my eyes out and trying to deal with disappointed parents, or Phill leaving me, or the loss of my first child. I shouldn't be here. This shouldn't be happening to me."

Jodi and I went for something to eat afterwards and had another serious conversation. I always end up feeling so guilty when I talk to anyone. I think the decision to place the baby for adoption is basically for Phill. I don't know if that's bad. I felt so lost when I got home, I cried and cried. I'm so scared about making a decision, and I don't know what to do about any of it.

Dear Journal,

Phill and I are having a hard time of this. We're both feeling lost and scared. He feels alone; I dread the future. He's overworked, tired, and stressed out about school, while I resent the fact that he's so busy we hardly see each other any more. It's all so hard, and I wonder when we will ever heal, or if we ever will. Is this roller coaster headed straight down, or is there light and hope at the end of this tunnel?

He's at home with his parents, and I'm here in the city. After a busy week of overtime, I'd like to stay home and do nothing tomorrow. But instead, Phill's mom and his sister Elizabeth are taking me shopping. They've offered to buy me some maternity clothes, which I really need right now. I appreciate it, but I'm just so tired. Maybe Phill will call me and say, "I'm picking you up, darling," and come to get me.

Problems with Adoption:

- Terrible guilt—am I doing the wrong thing? Everyone hurt (Mom and Dad)
- Having people talk/wonder/drive me insane
- Will not help or fix Phill's strained relationship with my family
- Depression—will I be all alone for months to heal? Will Phill be there as much as I need him?

- Will I resent Phill? Regret our decision?
- Will our relationship suffer/break?
- Will we feel supported?

Questions for Lauren:

- How do you feel about adoption now?
- Were you supported by your family/church?
- Did you grieve/need lots of time (how much?)/get depressed?
- How did the baby's father feel?
- Did your parents support you?
- Would you recommend ongoing contact with the baby?
- Did you bluntly tell everyone who asked what you had decided or play along with whatever they said?
- Did you feel guilty?
- How does it affect you now? Is this going to ruin my life?
- How did your relationship with your boyfriend change?
- Did he and your parents have a good relationship?
- What happens at the hospital?
- Can you give me any other advice?

Dear Journal,

Last night I went through a huge range of emotions. Jodi called me to say that she really thought I should ask my mom to be my labour coach. I guess she's had weird feelings of being "in the middle." I don't know how that would work, but maybe I'll talk to Mom about it anyway. Then I told Jodi about all the mixed-up feelings I've been having lately, and she reminded me of something very important: I need to make the decision that's right between God and me. That's the only way I'll ever feel peace about the whole thing. That statement stopped me in my tracks. It seems like lately I've forgotten that. But I still don't know what the right thing is, and I'm afraid I might run out of time before I know.

Phill called me after that and I was still crying. But we had an amazing talk, one I wish we could have had a long time ago, and I felt so much better afterwards. I was able to tell him all my fears, especially the ones regarding his relationship with my parents, and he was able to reassure me. He hasn't come over on the weekend for a long time, and I think that's put some unfriendly distance between them. He would like to make things right with Mom and Dad, and I was so happy to hear him say that.

I also expressed my concern about my recovery after I have the baby, how I'll need him so much but I'm afraid he'll be busy with school. He told me not to worry; if I need him, he'll be there. He also said that his priorities have been a little backwards lately, but I'm far more important to him than school and I should never think that he's too busy to talk to me. I felt amazing when we finally said good-bye. I was so relieved to have my Phill back.

I had another doctor's appointment this morning. Dr. Michiko said the baby's getting quite big; another inch of growth and he'll be under my ribs. Next month is my last monthly appointment; then I'll start going every two weeks. When I told Caroline at work about the baby being so big, she said he's probably going to get too big for me and I'll end up having a C-section. That's fine with me, as long as they schedule it ahead of time and not after twenty-four hours of unproductive labour!

Dear Journal,

I feel better mentally today. Mom called me last night, and I keep thinking how stressed she sounded on the phone. She actually asked me if I think everything is going to work out between me and Phill in the end. I don't even feel like phoning her again. Does she have that little faith in us? Poor Mom. I wish I could understand her and relieve her fears.

Dear Journal,

Phill's been so sweet lately, it's wonderful. He's meeting my family with me for lunch tomorrow, which I'm glad about. He hasn't wanted to see them in a long time. I'm so proud of him. He's really making an effort to mend things, when it should probably be my parents making the first move.

He got to feel our baby move today. I was really excited. Usually when someone puts their hand on my stomach, the baby holds perfectly still until they go away. He must know who his daddy is.

Dear Journal,

I spent the afternoon at Phill's today, just watching TV and talking. I'm confused again. He said he's been thinking about lots of things lately. I think he's been having second thoughts again about adoption. I sometimes wonder if he will end up changing his mind. But in saying that, does it not indicate that I want to keep this baby and I'd only be giving it up for Phill? I keep thinking that I shouldn't block out the idea of keeping him, that I should think out all my options. The way Phill and I love each other now, how could he leave if I kept the baby? Is that the basis of my whole decision? I'm beginning to doubt all the things I thought I had decided before. But what would happen if I kept him? The only thing I know is that I'd move home. What about Phill? Would we continue dating? Would he come to love this baby? Would people, including my parents, think less of him and begin to leave him out of the picture? Would he finish school? What about my job and my apartment?

Everyone around me, my family, and the people at church, say they'd support me, but I don't think they even know the meaning of the word. The only "support" a lot of people would give me is to say they're happy that I kept the baby. No matter how much "support" I'd have, no support would matter as much to me as Phill's, and even then it would still be just me dealing with everything.

Dear Journal,

Last night I got on my knees to pray and just began to cry. But I realized that I've forgotten that God is almighty and all powerful. He can change the hearts of man, and for Him nothing is impossible. I need to wait for Him, hope, trust, pray, and have patience. It's so hard to do. I find it nearly impossible.

Dear Journal,

Another emotional evening where nothing makes sense and Phill has no time for me. Not that it's his fault. I think I need to talk to Lauren and ask her all my questions.

Phill's going to try to find some time to sit down with me and have a big talk. Then, when his exams are done, we'll go to the adoption agency. Why does no one understand me? Or is it me that doesn't understand them?

Dear Journal,

This baby situation is plaguing me. I feel sorry for the baby. He didn't ask to be here, and nothing is his fault. I feel so guilty thinking about adoption, but it's the only way I see things working out. Sometimes I really wish that I could sit down here and write, "I'm keeping my baby." Then at least I could name him, teach him things, and pay for his piano lessons. I know that in ten years when I look back, I won't regret it or feel bad about doing it. The reason I feel bad now is Phill. What would he do and where would our relationship go? I know that countless people would tell me, "You shouldn't do anything because of him." But he is a huge part of my life; how can he not be a huge part of my decision? Everyone tries to tell me that he doesn't matter, and then I doubt or mistrust their advice. This baby is just as much his as mine. I feel like I'm running out of time and everything is getting harder.

Dear Journal,

I had an encouraging talk with Phill. He talked to his dad this evening about everything, and what he had to say was interesting and encouraging. His dad isn't opposed to adoption and is trying to have an open mind. I'm really glad about that and that they could talk about it. I feel better about things now, that someday everything will be okay and we will make it through this together even though it's hard. I wish my parents were easier to talk to. Maybe they are and I'm just too afraid to try.

Dear Journal,

I've been doing a lot of thinking since last night, and I'm beginning to realize that I am influenced greatly by what other people think. The fact that Phill's dad is open to adoption made the idea of adoption seem so much brighter and better. I think the only thing standing in the way of me having peace about adoption is that other people make me feel guilty about it. If I knew that my parents supported me and were really trying to understand Phill and me, it would be so much easier to deal with. I would feel free to talk to them; maybe Mom would be my confidante instead of Caroline or Karen or Marianne or Jodi. I feel guilty about going against them. But I keep praying for them.

Dear Journal,

I feel like I haven't seen or talked to Phill for an eternity, and the prospect of a whole weekend without him seems grim. Poor guy. No one ever really believes me at church when I tell them he's not there because he's busy with homework or school. Maybe they don't want to believe it. I just talked to him on the phone and he's so busy, I won't be able to see him all next week, either! I miss him so much. I'm always torn between trying to understand his busy schedule and wanting him to make time for me. But I just can't do that to him.

Dear Journal,

Today I read this entire journal, and although I still felt some unease about some of the questions I've written down, I felt more confidence than ever about adoption. It's still scary, and it will still be hard, but I think we will be able to feel confident about that decision, especially if we have other people's support.

Dear Journal,

Mom picked me up this afternoon and we went shopping. We had coffee at a café, and while we were there, she asked me quite casually if we had decided what to do with the baby. So I told her, fearfully. She didn't freak out (why was I expecting her to?). I know it was hard for her, but all she said was that if I did still decide to keep him, they would help any way they could. She also commented that this should be the happiest time of my life, the birth of my first child, but it's been nothing like that. I feel better that she knows. I've wanted to tell her for weeks, but I just couldn't. I've been too scared. Even today, I really wanted to say more about how we've struggled for weeks with this dilemma and how I was so afraid of disappointing them, but no words would come. I really wish she would have asked me how I feel about it and helped me to talk about it. I wish I could tell her about my feelings and thoughts without always being so concerned about what she and Dad will think of me. I want them to be concerned about how I'm doing, not just about the final decision. But I do feel better knowing that we've made a decision. I can focus on it, instead of it plaguing me.

December

Dear Journal,

I looked back at the list entitled "Problems with Adoption" that I made a month ago and none of the issues I listed seem like real threats any more. I guess we've come a long way since the beginning of this pregnancy.

Today I called the adoption agency and made an appointment with a lady named Leah for Phill and me, now that he's on Christmas break from school. She is an adoption counsellor and she seemed very nice so I think things will go well, as long as neither of us freaks out. Actually I'm looking forward to having my questions answered and having a clearer picture of what things will be like.

I called the unemployment office, too. I only need to have worked 600 hours in the last year to qualify for maternity benefits, and I get fifteen weeks paid time off if I give the baby up. Every time I write that phrase I inwardly cringe, thinking that if my son or daughter ever read these words it would sound so cold and uncaring. But I do care about my baby; I want the best for it and I really hope things work out.

"As for me, I will call upon God; and the LORD shall save me. Evening, and morning, and at noon, will I pray, and cry aloud: and he shall hear my voice. He hath delivered my soul

in peace from the battle that was against me: for there were many with me." (Psalm 55:16-18).

Return unto thy rest, O my soul; for the LORD hath dealt bountifully with thee. For thou hast delivered my soul from death, mine eyes from tears, and my feet from falling. I will walk before the LORD in the land of the living (Psalm 116:7-9).

Dear Journal,

I've been getting some Christmas cards in the mail, and I received one from Lucy, the lady I spoke to at the Pregnancy Crisis Centre a few months ago. For some reason, that card is my favourite. It has a very simple message; she just wished Phill and me a Merry Christmas, but in some way it makes me feel safe to look at it. Maybe it's because she included Phill in the greeting, or maybe it's just because she remembered me and cared enough to send me a card. It makes me feel a little more hopeful to know that someone out there thinks that we'll make it and is praying for us.

Dear Journal,

Suddenly it's very late and I'm tired. I had a hard time again last night. James came over and we watched a movie. Before he left, we talked a bit about serious things and he said some stuff about my situation that hurt. Like, Mom will be devastated if I give up the baby, and everyone wants me to keep it. So I called Phill and cried to him for awhile. He always makes me feel better.

We went to our appointment today at the adoption agency. It went really well. Our counsellor, Leah, is really nice. She explained all the steps of the adoption process to us and got us started on the first one: application forms. Both of us felt really good when we left.

Dear Journal,

Phill called me. He is such an amazing boy. He wants very much to take care of me and is happy about the way I count on him and need him so much. He's very confident about our decision. We talked a little bit more about names and such and that right after I deliver in the hospital, both of us want it to be just the two of us there for awhile. He talked to Marianne about David and Beth, and even though they have no clue that we have them in mind, they already have all kinds of baby stuff.

I had a good talk with Jo, too. She's been very understanding and supportive. She said she's already made plans with a friend to drive into the city from school to see me when I have the baby. All of my teachers know, and they're all praying for us. I'm so relieved and glad about that. I was worried about their reactions should I show up at Jo's Christmas concert next week looking very pregnant.

He will fulfil the desire of them that fear him: he also will hear their cry, and will save them. (Psalm 145:19).

Dear Journal,

It hasn't been the greatest day. Last night Phill picked me up and I stayed the night at his place. This morning we went to our appointment at the agency. It was tough. We watched a video that made us realize just how tough adoption will be. Talking later, Phill said that he's unsure about deciding. He thinks different ways at different times. It feels like we've hit another wall. We're back to wondering which decision to make, instead of moving ahead. But we got a bunch of forms to fill out about decision-making, and I'd like to do them together. Our next appointment is January 10.

Dear Journal,

I feel absolutely massive. I see Jo and the other girls at church and get so envious. They don't have this big uncomfortable ball attached to them or chunky thighs or a butt that sticks out! Sometimes even now, I feel so ashamed of my belly. I want to hide it, but it's impossible since I'm already eight months along. I keep thinking that this should not be happening to me. I've known for six months and still I think that way.

When I think about parenting and the responsibilities, work, and busyness, I honestly don't want to do it. I don't want to deal with it or even attempt to handle it. I feel selfish and guilty for thinking that way, but it's the truth. I do love my baby and I know I wouldn't regret parenting, but I don't at all want to do it alone. I really want to sit down with Phill and go through all the papers we got and just discuss everything.

Dear Journal,

I went through the forms from the agency on decision-making, but the questions are hard to answer. I'd really like to do them with Phill one day. Mom and I talked a bit about it this evening. She sounded like she knew for sure that we would be placing. But she said no matter what the pros and cons are, if we really want to do something, nothing's impossible. Will my parents then assume we don't want our child if we place it? Is adoption completely selfish in our position? Phill called me in the evening. We didn't have too much to say. I'm really dreading when he goes back to school. When will we have time for everything? How is he going to handle it all? The other night we talked about marriage. It was fun to talk about, but who knows when it will happen, especially in light of what we're facing now. Sometimes it makes me sad because my wedding daydreams may not come true. Everything is up in the air. Everything is hard. I still have so many doubts and questions.

Dear Journal,

Last night was Jo's Christmas concert and I did end up going. I felt so self-conscious, but no one looked at me funny or said anything. In fact, the only comment I got the whole evening was from a guy I graduated with who told me I looked really big. I never really liked him, and I found his comment very rude. You don't say that kind of thing to a pregnant girl! I felt like hitting him, but of course I didn't. Besides that, everything went fine.

Dear Journal,

I can't even celebrate Christmas Day in peace. My uncle told me a story after the church service this morning about his fifteen-year-old niece who got pregnant and kept the baby. This girl later said that it was the best decision she'd ever made. That's nice, I thought. Good for her. But then it made me think: will my church family support and love me if I place our baby for adoption, or is their support conditional on what the outcome is? In other words, are they only going to support me if I keep it? That sounds awfully shallow, but not once has anyone said to me that they'll support me no matter what I decide.

Dear Journal,

Am I going to make it through the postpartum days after delivery and adoption? I can see myself just sitting around, not doing anything—because I won't feel like doing anything—and getting more and more upset at being all alone. What am I going to do to overcome all the depression? I'm afraid. Delivery and placing the baby is one thing, but what about later?

Dear Journal,

Last night Phill and I had a really good talk on the phone. He asks how the baby is doing every time we talk. In all our talk of adoption, the thing that makes me cry most is hearing Phill say that he loves the baby. Tears of happiness. And I know he really does. I don't know how it happened. Maybe it only started when he first felt the baby moving. But now he asks how the baby is as much as he asks me how I am. What a long way we've come.

January

Dear Journal,

I'm sick of letting people down! I'm sick of writing unhappy and negative things in this journal. I'm sick of feeling like I'm doing what someone else thinks is wrong. I called Jodi this evening and everything was fine until she asked me what we had decided. I guess she wasn't prepared for the answer, as she got really upset. Maybe she needs time to deal with it and get used to it, but her response really scared me. How can she be my labour coach if she thinks I'm doing something wrong? I'm sick of thinking about all the other people who are going to respond the same way. So I called Phill and, as he always does, he made me feel better. He said it's unfair that people around me think I'm made of steel and can handle anything they say to me. Why do they think that I need their opinion on top of everything else?

Dear Journal,

Phill and I have been talking so well lately. I feel like our communication has improved so much over the last few months. We tell each other everything about how we think and feel. He's such a great guy, so smart, sensitive and realistic.

Dear Journal,

I've had a terrible evening. My grandma phoned and said a bunch of things regarding our decision about the baby that really hurt me. I don't want to write what she said, because then I'd remember it. First I called Phill, because I always call him when I'm crying. Then I called James to see if we could do something this evening and get me out of this apartment, but he had already gone out. So I talked to his roommate, who also gave me his opinion about our situation. After his fifteen-minute long speech, he said, "But whatever you decide to do, I'll still support you." What a load of crap! That doesn't erase the fact that I know I'd be disappointing him and everyone else. What do these people think *support* actually means? So many people have said they'll support me, but all they've really done is tell me what they think I should do. There have been very few people who have expressed genuine concern for me as a person and not just as a topic of gossip. One Sunday, a cousin of mine came up to me and said that if I ever needed to talk or if I wanted to come over for supper any time, I could. I appreciated that offer more than I let on at the time. That's the kind of support I need. I don't want people to care about the final outcome only. Why can't they care about me? I think after all of this is over, if it ever is, I'm going to erase the word "support" from my vocabulary. I'm sick of hearing it from people who don't mean it!

Everything I've been told has thrown me into a huge inner turmoil, filled with questions I can't answer. I've been crying for two hours and trying to write down my thoughts. I need someone to talk to, but there's no one I can call. I tried calling one of my aunts to get Lauren's phone number but she wasn't home, so I left a message.

No matter how much adversity I face or how lost and hopeless I feel, there it is in front of me all the time: adoption. I keep returning to it. Why? Because it's peaceful, relieving, loving and solving? Or because I'm selfish and running away? How can we make a final decision if we can't answer these kinds of questions?

Dear Journal,

I saw Phill this afternoon. He is sick and didn't go to school, but he needed to get out of his apartment, so he came over. He is such a source of comfort to me. He is the one person in my life who understands and sticks by me. All of his words and actions have me in mind, even when he feels awful. It was so comforting to have his head in my lap, his cheek against the baby, me stroking his hair. I love him to pieces, and I don't know how I could do this without him.

Dear Journal,

Well, I finally got enough courage to call Lauren. It was amazing talking to someone who's been there and can tell you a bit of what it's like. I hope I can remember all the things she said:

- Everything is based on your attitude and how you look at things
- I will need everyone in that delivery room to be completely supportive of our decision and not try to sway me
- Adoption is and can be wonderful; Lauren said she has no regrets
- It's very hard to make the decision and go through with it but it's also the best decision you'll ever make
- Everyone thinks it's so wonderful that a couple can adopt a child, so why can't it be wonderful that a teenage girl allows that to happen?
- Everyone may be against you now, but everyone heals over time
- You come to a point where you have to disregard what other people think and do what you have to do

- Lauren thinks we'll be fine because we're thinking so positively
- Every day gets easier, but the first year is the hardest
- Yes, you will think about that child every day, but you can think of good things, not bad
- Contact with the baby and the adoptive family, in the first while, you have to play by ear
- Don't let anyone in the hospital say, "Let's just take him home." You don't need or want to hear that
- Holding the baby is definitely a good idea
- Relationships with friends and family during pregnancy may have been awful but are stronger and better than ever later on (in Lauren's experience)
- Answer honestly anyone who questions you; ask them, "If you couldn't have kids, wouldn't you want someone to let you be a mom?"

It was extremely encouraging to talk to her and has given me that renewed hope I needed. She answered my questions and gave me all the helpful information she could think of. She didn't once comment on our decision, whether it's right or wrong. I'm so grateful for that. She said I could call her any time, and I think I will if more questions arise.

Dear Journal,

I'm still thinking and worrying about what Grandma and James's roommate said to me yesterday. To be honest, I've been having doubts about adoption even though I think it's the best thing to do. I've been worrying about everyone around me, how most of them will never understand or even try to understand. What kinds of things are they going to say to me? No matter how many times I've been told not to worry about what other people say, I just can't stop caring. These are people who matter, like my grandma, my church family... and I don't want to live at odds with everyone for the rest of my life.

Phill is still sick. I feel tired... tired of working, thinking, getting up early. I need to get this all over with and move on to the next chapter of my life.

Dear Journal,

I've had a hard day. Physically, I've been hot, very tired, and one of my ribs is aching badly. Emotionally, I am drained. Phill and I spent two and a half hours at the agency this morning talking to Leah about grief, stress and all the things playing into our situation. Then we looked at files, including David and Beth's, and another couple whom we know. Their names are Keith and Lisa, the same couple that Lauren gave her baby boy to five years ago. Keith was also one of our high-school teachers. We are now considering both couples, but there are a lot of things to consider.

I talked to Mom, among other people, tonight. I told her about some of the things I'm going through, especially about the comments from other people that upset me, and I'm glad I finally got some of my feelings across. I've wanted to talk to her like this for a long time. But I also told her, when she asked me, that I do want to place our baby, that I'm not just going along with what Phill wants. I felt absolutely horrible and guilty, because I know what her opinion is about it. I love my parents dearly, and I feel more awful than there are words for, now that they know our decision. But why can't they ever leave that part of it alone? Why don't they ever just listen to how I'm feeling and forget about always reminding me that there is a decision to be made? I guess it's because they're my parents and they feel they have to guide me and talk about the hard things. It gets so tiring for me. It makes me not want to tell them anything because they don't ever listen without putting their two cents in.

It's everyone else's opinions that make it most difficult for me. It hurts me to know that I am hurting so many others. That one simple fact is what makes our situation so trying and so impossible.

Dear Journal,

Jo was in the city today so she picked me up and took me home to Mom and Dad's for the weekend. We had a really good talk about adoption. She thinks that Keith and Lisa are a good choice. I'm beginning to think that David and Beth are a bit too close, since Marianne and her husband see them often. What if someday their son and our son get to talking and he finds out that his friend's Uncle Phill and Auntie Erin are really his parents? I'm trying to think of what is best for our baby.

Dear Journal,

Something amazing has happened today. God has heard my prayer and answered it in a wonderful way. I have the full support of my parents! This morning we sat down at the table to talk, and they began asking questions about our adoption plans and appointments. As we continued talking, I learned that they agree with our decision and believe as we do that adoption is the best choice for the baby. They believe the Lord has led us to this decision—all of us, not just Phill and I—and think that Keith and Lisa are an excellent choice for parents for our baby. They would be very comfortable with us choosing them. I am so happy about the things they said. Dad also encouraged me not to let what other people say get to me.

It was such a huge relief to connect with Mom and Dad like this. Dad said if people we think are important say we've made the wrong decision, stop listening to them. If God has led us to this decision, no one else's opinion should matter. I'm happier than I can say.

The rest of my day has been uneventful and relaxing. I called Phill in the evening. He was very happy to hear about the talk I had with Mom and Dad. He also said that our prayers have been answered. I told him that I was really leaning toward Keith and Lisa now and he said that was fine. My reasons are all based on what I think would be best for our baby. He would have an older brother, since they have already adopted one child, and there would be less chance of an awkward situation between our child and his biological relatives. Phill really likes the idea of our baby having a sibling. Mom and Dad are really glad about Keith and Lisa, too. It's strange how God leads us to where we are to go, although nothing's final yet. We hope to go back to the agency on Thursday.

I think we're going to keep who we're giving our baby to very confidential, since not everyone needs to know while Jo is still attending school where Keith is teaching. I'd hate for kids to come up to her and make comments about their baby being her niece or nephew.

I read back in this journal and it's amazing to see all the milestones we've reached and all the troubles we've overcome: we've made a decision, Phill and I both love our baby, Phill's parents and my parents get along well, my parents support us, we've chosen an excellent family... it's exciting to see God work in our lives.

Dear Journal,

Phill and I went to the adoption agency this morning. We basically just told Leah that we have chosen a family and we would like to have a meeting with them. So she got on the phone and called Keith and Lisa. They weren't home at the time so she called me later at work. She had talked with Lisa who said they'd be excited to meet with us! So we're getting together with them on Tuesday at 2:00 p.m. I'm actually really excited.

One of the things I'm supposed to do as part of the adoption process is write my baby a letter that he'll read later in life. I worked on that this evening. It's so hard to explain things in one page of loose-leaf; hard to put together nine months of struggle to try to make him understand.

Dear Journal,

Work is getting so hard! Today I was seriously considering leaving early. It seemed so impossible to do anything. I'm just so thankful that the girl I work with on evenings offered to do all the sweeping and mopping at the end of the night.

Phill called me at work today. He's so frustrated with school that he's about ready to give up. It seems that this semester he just can't seem to get any information to stick in his head. I wish there was some way I could help him.

And Uncle Henry called me this evening. He and Aunt Kate want to come visit me in the near future. I get so frustrated with them. What are they planning on doing? Do they think they are going to make me change my mind because adoption's not what they want me to do? Maybe it won't be so bad and I shouldn't jump to conclusions, but I'm afraid. Isn't it awful how you come to mistrust people that you should be able to trust the most, just because of a misunderstanding or bad experience? That's how I feel now about my own pastor; yet, they're my aunt and uncle, too. It's twice as bad because they're family. I'm scared of them. I have a feeling that when they come over they will only make me feel worse. But I won't let them guilt me into anything. They're coming on Monday.

Dear Journal,

This whole Monday visit thing is really scaring me. Phill thinks I should phone them back and tell them not to come if they don't have anything positive or supportive to say to me. But

I don't think I can do that. This is such a ridiculously delicate situation because not only is Uncle Henry the leading pastor at church, he's a relative, family friend, and I know his visits are out of genuine concern. They think of me almost as a daughter. I think I will just have to let them come over, hear what they have to say, and tell them gently but honestly what I think and feel. If what they have to say is negative, I'll just thank them for their opinion and tell them that we've already made our decision, one that is well thought out, prayed about, and that both of our families support. What more can I do? Sometimes I'd like to think that I don't deserve this, but you have to live with the consequences of your sin, and that includes hard things like this. Maybe deep down inside I'm hoping that Phill's prayer for a miracle will be answered and they'll turn out to be encouraging instead of discouraging.

Tomorrow at work I want to talk to Caroline about how my hours are getting too long and how difficult I'm finding it. Maybe we can work something out.

Dear Journal,

I have one more week of work left, and I don't know if I will survive it. Whereas yesterday wasn't too bad, today was awful. I went home at lunch because I felt so useless. Everything is sore, I can't walk properly, there is tons of pressure on the bottom of my belly, and I feel like I have to pee every half-hour. I thought these things were characteristic of the baby dropping, but he hasn't moved. He's still jammed up under my ribs. I took it easy all afternoon, but I'm not looking forward to going to bed. I'll probably be up all night, sore and uncomfortable. I want to wake up tomorrow and see this kid farther down! For whatever reason, he likes to sit very high up, right at the bottom of my rib cage and mostly on the left side. His pushing is beginning to hurt.

Dear Journal,

I've had a terrible last few nights and days, including this one. The pain in my hips, back, and lower abdomen got worse over the weekend, keeping me up all night last night (and now), preventing me from going to church, and finally pushing me to tears.

Phill was over Sunday afternoon. He got me to call my doctor, but she is on holidays or something; then he took me to the city when I couldn't bear it at home any more. We decided to go to emergency, so we went to the hospital. They hooked me up to fetal monitors and did all sorts of stuff. There was a possibility that I was in early labour, but because I'm only thirty-five-weeks pregnant, which is five weeks early, they'd have to send me to another hospital. So off we went and the same procedures were done there. This doctor, whom I really didn't like, determined that I was not in labour but have a urinary tract infection. So he prescribed some antibiotics, which we picked up on the way back to my apartment.

Phill was so good to me. He hadn't eaten any supper and had a headache, but he was calm and supportive, rubbing my back and telling me I was doing good. And now here I am, at 1:30 a.m. My back hurts enough to prevent me from sleeping at all. It's so awful having to stay up all night in pain. I don't know what to do with myself. I had a long hot shower before, which seemed to help, but I'm not allowed to have a bath, because of the infection.

Mom is coming in to see me tomorrow. She called Uncle Henry for me and told them not to come over because of all this. Is this our answer to prayer?

I'll be off work at least two days, so I may as well quit now altogether, since I only had this week left anyway. I called Caroline once this weekend and I'll call her again tomorrow.

The medication is supposed to kick in within twenty-four to forty-eight hours. So I suppose I have all night and all tomorrow like this. I'm so tired, though. I wish I could sleep.

I guess there are some good things about our whole hospital escapade. I found out the baby is in the right position, head down, and that his head is right up against my cervix. So it won't be long now anyways.

Dear Journal,

I'm really not sure how I'm going to survive this. And I have to deliver a baby at the end? Forget it! This is too much pain. I was up until 5:00 this morning. I just about went out of my mind. I called Mom at 4:30 a.m. and she told me to load up on Tylenol. So that's what I did, and I ended up sleeping for two hours. I got up for breakfast at 7:30 and have been trying to find ways to pass the time ever since. Showers are nice, but my skin is beginning to get really raw and dry from them since I've had so many. Every time I sit down, my eyes close and I want so much to sleep, but if I lie down I don't get more than fifteen minutes before my back hurts so much I can't sleep any more and I have to get up.

Dear Journal,

This day has felt like the equivalent of three days. It goes so slowly, always with severe hip and lower back pain threatening me. I'm beginning to wonder if these pains really have anything to do with the infection itself, or if they are a constant part of being close to labour. I just want relief! I am terrified of another night like last night.

Mom came for lunch and took me shopping. The rest of the day has been boring. I don't know what I can do with myself that won't hurt. With all of the signs I've been having, I could go into labour today or next week, according to all my books. I called Mom and she recommended calling my doctor to tell her all my troubles and ask what the procedure is for going to the hospital and such, and also to pack my bag and be ready to go. Yikes, she sounded serious. But I am so ready to have this baby, anything to get out of another unproductive, sleepless night. I've paged Dr. Michiko and am awaiting a call back. I guess I should pack my stuff.

Dr. M just called me back, and it was sort of an unsatisfying, typical phone call that made me feel like my questions were dumb. She always makes me feel that way. I didn't even want to call her. But she told me that the bottom line is, if I'm concerned, I don't need to phone first, I just go to the appropriate hospital. They can't diagnose over the phone, so I'd have to be seen anyway. Great. This stinks.

Dear Journal,

So much has happened in the last few days; it's all very hard to believe. Monday night, the last time I wrote, I ended up trying to time my contractions to see if they really had a pattern, but they didn't. I called Mom a second time because I just couldn't stand the pain, and she told me to call the hospital and speak to a nurse there. I did that and the nurse told me to take some Tylenol, wait an hour, and call back if there was no improvement. I called her back in half an hour. I was getting desperate. She told me that, if I wanted to be seen, I'd have to go to a different hospital, because their ward was full and they might be closing it, but to check with my doctor on where I should go.

Well, I didn't think my doctor would care, but I paged her anyway at 3:00 a.m. and called Phill. Dr. M wasn't helpful at all, saying to just go anywhere. So Phill came and picked me up and we went to another hospital. This was the third one I'd been to! Again I was hooked up to monitors and everything and a really nice doctor came in and asked a whole bunch of questions, but in the end, all he determined was that it was all due to my infection and I'd just have to live with the pain until the medication kicked in. And it probably also had to do with my joints loosening and all that last-month-of-pregnancy stuff. I was very disappointed. Poor Phill had been up all night again for me, and we had come for nothing. Phill dropped me off at 6:00 a.m. and I actually slept for a few hours.

The morning was really nice. The pain subsided and I went to the grocery store with Karen. When Phill got out of school at 1:00, he came by and we left for the adoption agency. It was our meeting with Keith and Lisa. By that time the pain was returning, but I thought I could handle it. The meeting went well. Keith and Lisa were very laid back and we got a lot of details worked out, "just in case," I told them. I had to leave the room twice because my back pain was so severe. I'd go to the bathroom down the hall and contort in agony until it subsided and I could join the meeting again.

We talked a bit about names. They like Julia, Kate, and Samantha for a girl, but were stuck on the name Joshua for a boy. I'm not crazy about that name, but they're the ones who have to call him that forever. We left around 5:00. I was supposed to go to my aunt's for supper with James and some other people, but I didn't want to cause a scene by leaving the table in pain every five minutes.

I paced around my apartment the whole evening, which seemed to help. It was the only thing that kept me sane, walking in a circle through the kitchen, around the dining room table, and back through the living room. I looked at every list in every book I have, comparing real labour versus false labour, but I seemed to be having signs of both. I even called Phill's mom, who used to be a nurse, to see what she thought. There was no way I wanted to make another hospital visit at night for nothing. So I determined that no matter what, if there was no pattern to the pain, I would stay home.

However, by the time my roommates went to bed, I was really desperate. I cried constantly, partly from pain, but mostly from frustration and exhaustion. I called Mom and told her I couldn't take it any more. She didn't know what to do or say. But I was at the end of my rope. If I wasn't in labour—and I was sure I wasn't—then what was causing such agonizing pain? After we hung up, with once again no solution, I took another shower, but it didn't help much. When I got out, Karen said someone had called for me from triage at the hospital we had been at the night before. I called back right away and spoke with Paul, a nurse there. He was very nice, said he had spoken to my mom and thought I should come in. He thought maybe my antibiotics weren't working and I might have to stay overnight on an IV. I was so relieved to have some kind of an answer. I called Phill and packed my bag.

He picked me up at 11:00 p.m. I started to say I was sorry for keeping him up again when he had classes to go to in the morning, but he said he didn't want to hear a word about it. When the pain got really bad, he reminded me to breathe through it.

Paul was waiting for us at the hospital and put us in a room right away. Another doctor came in and began asking questions. He was really nice and asked me if they had done a pelvic exam the night before. When I said no, he thought they had better. He did it right away, and when it was done, he said, "Well, we're going to have this baby tonight." I stared at him as he told me that I was already between seven and eight centimetres dilated. All I could say was, "Holy cow."

Phill went to call my parents, and I was hooked up to an IV and some monitors. Phill came back and sat beside me, held my hand, and helped me breathe through contractions, which were suddenly developing a pattern now (how convenient). For an inexperienced and untrained labour coach, Phill was excellent. He said and did all the things they taught us in prenatal classes—and he didn't even go to any. When my parents arrived, I had Mom on one side and Phill on the other. They told me it was too late for an epidural or Demerol but I could have laughing gas. The contractions were pretty strong, but I thought I could handle them, so I refused. I was mostly afraid of having a mask over my face and breathing warm, stinky gas. I didn't want to be any more uncomfortable than I already was! At 2:00 a.m., I was told it was time to push. Phill left, and I didn't know until later that he sat right outside the door and listened to the whole delivery!

At 3:52 a.m., a boy was born. My first thoughts were that he had a nice cry and that he looked big. They put him in an incubator beside my bed, and we watched them clean him up. Mom was very excited; I just couldn't believe that he was the same thing that had been kicking me all those months. He had fuzzy black hair and dark blue eyes.

Phill and Dad came back in, and we all just looked at him for a bit; then my parents went home. Phill sat with me and held my hand for awhile. I was so exhausted, I fell asleep between sentences. He told me that he really admired me for what I had just gone through. Then he went home to sleep but told me that he'd skip classes that day and be back in the afternoon. Our baby was weighed at six pounds, eight ounces and measured about twenty and one-half inches. Paul came in after awhile to take me up to a different room. There I tried to sleep.

After lunch, the hospital social worker came to talk to me. We had a good long talk. I still felt the same about adoption. I hadn't changed my mind or gone through any huge emotional turmoil like we had been warned about. Phill arrived at 2:00 and we had our baby brought to us for about an hour and a half. I had bottle-fed and held him already that morning. He's such a good baby. I haven't heard him cry since delivery. He just sleeps all the time. He's very cute. He's so little and has all this fuzzy, spiky hair. He's got really long fingers and big feet.

Phill had already called Keith and Lisa, who sounded pretty excited. He had also called Leah. She's coming to talk with me this morning. All sorts of people visited me yesterday. Most of Phill's family came, bringing gifts and everything. My family came, too, in the evening. After everyone left, Phill climbed into bed with me. We shut off the lights and talked quietly. We're both happy—happy about our baby, happy about our decision, happy with Keith and Lisa. Everything about this pregnancy, labour, and afterwards has been so opposite of what was expected.

Dear Journal,

This morning Leah came to see me, and I spent some time with the baby. I gave him a bath, changed him, and fed him. Phill has been doing a lot of thinking and has been re-considering our options. He told me he's not changing his mind, but he said, if this wasn't an open adoption, he wouldn't be able to do it. I've had some confusing thoughts myself. The fact that the baby is going with Keith and Lisa tomorrow sort of scares me, but, at the same time, I'll be honestly relieved. I feel very inadequate, unprepared, and not ready to care for a baby. I'm not even sure how I feel about thinking that way.

I didn't get a break this afternoon. Mom and Dad stopped in. We went to the nursery to see the baby. Dad didn't say much the whole time. He didn't even want to hold him. It made me feel awful. This is probably very hard for them.

Phill's mom and Elizabeth also came. His mom was so excited about the baby. She fed him and played with him. Seeing how enthused she was is hard to deal with. She said, if we kept the baby, it would work out; they'd help us any way they could. I understand where she's coming from, but it still made me feel bad. What am I supposed to say to comments like that?

Jodi and her husband came after that. She was very emotional, and the first thing she said was, "Why don't you just take him home?" I didn't know what to say, and then she quickly added, "Or shouldn't I ask that?" I told her no, she shouldn't. I understand her comment as well, but as I lay in bed waiting for Phill, I felt really miserable. I wondered if there was something wrong with me, if I was a horrible person. Tomorrow we get discharged and are meeting Keith and Lisa to give the baby to them. They are calling him Joshua.

Dear Journal,

Yesterday was a hard day. First thing in the morning, Phill got a phone call from his dad, who said some very mean things to him. Then the lawyer came to the hospital with papers for us to sign. After that, we spent the morning in my bed, talking and crying.

Leah came at 11:30. We dressed and fed little Joshua, packed up our stuff, and went to meet Keith and Lisa. We spent a lot of time there by ourselves and with Leah, trying to sort out our thoughts, feelings, and reasons for what we were doing. We were having a hard time with the last one. With our little baby sleeping on our laps, anything seemed possible. But really, nothing has changed. We decided it was the wrong time to be thinking about this, so we left Joshua with them, knowing that we would visit them on Sunday. We walked out the door holding hands and feeling okay about what we were doing.

Mom called me in the evening. I could tell that she was hurting, and she said things to me that hurt me. She said that Joshua is the most beautiful baby she's ever seen and that she fell in love with him as soon as she saw him. She told me to keep re-considering because it would work to keep him. That was really hard to hear. It makes me doubt our decision and really wonder if it would work. It's so hard to predict how we're going to feel about this in a year or two. It tears me apart to keep bouncing back between the two options. We have three weeks to change our minds. Keith told us not to worry about them, just to figure things out for ourselves and do what we think is best for us.

Dear Journal,

I'm feeling a little afraid. I called home and talked to Jo. She's finished her exams and is home for the week. It sounds like my parents have been moping around the house and saying all kinds of things. Jo is really sick of it. She said she yelled at Mom once and is dying to go back to school to get away from them. I feel so awful about how my family is coming apart at the seams. If only I could bear the weight alone instead of having it affect the people I love most. I'm afraid that we're just going to gang up on each other at a time when we all need each other the most.

I called Lauren again and had a really good talk with her. Basically, she said what deep down I already knew: things are going to be crazy for awhile. I have to give things time and talk to my family honestly about my feelings. She said that my mom is probably thinking with her heart and not her head, which is to be expected, and I understand. The next few weeks are going to be really hard, and we just have to remind ourselves that this is what we've decided, we're happy and okay with it, and all those other opinions are coming from people who are not in our shoes and never will be.

Dear Journal,

I sit here in total disbelief. The events of the past two days have been horrifying and wonderful. Throughout this pregnancy, I have been praying for a miracle, and today Jesus made the miracle happen.

Sunday was an awful day. Phill picked me up at my apartment at 12:00, and we went to my grandma's for lunch, along with my family and some of my aunts. After dinner was over, Dad began to talk and cry, telling us that they think adoption is wrong and that we should keep our baby at all costs. I've never seen my dad cry like that. So everything they told us before about adoption being the best choice was not true any more.

We left there, with me crying as usual, and went to visit Keith, Lisa, and Joshua. That was the best part of the day. Everything was comfortable and fine. We talked to them quite a bit about what we were going through. Of course, they couldn't offer any advice, but they listened and sympathized.

From there we drove to Phill's parents' place and had supper. After the meal was over, Phill's dad started his talk with us. It was the most horrifying thing I have ever had to go through. He hadn't slept in three nights and was telling us about all these visions he'd had. He insulted and attacked Phill directly, over and over. He blamed him and him alone for everything that was happening. He said Satan was in him. I cried and cried because of all the things he was saying, but then he blamed Phill for that, too. We couldn't say anything that he would listen to or that made sense to him. So we just sat there and took it. Phill's mom didn't say anything the entire time either. In the end, Phill's dad wanted me to stay behind to talk while Phill went back to the city, but there was no way I wanted to do that, and thank God, Phill refused to leave without me. I had a terrible headache and I was bawling, and I just didn't think I could handle any more. I was worried that I might hemorrhage from stress. Finally, the only thing I could muster was a tiny voice that said, "I want to go home." Phill took my hand and got up to leave, but his dad tried to physically separate us and stop us, until Phill's mom intervened. She took me to the entrance to get my stuff, and I couldn't see what was happening between Phill and his dad. I had this terrible thought that he was going to hit Phill.

We did finally get out of there, both of us crying. I was terrified. We drove back to the city. Phill had been afraid his dad might have taken his truck keys so we couldn't get away. It was so terrible. By the time we reached home, we were again trying to think positively and thought that we should sit down together and really think through our reasons and what would, or could, happen if we got our baby back. If his dad was trying to change our minds about giving up our baby, he went about it all the wrong way. I don't know why he didn't even try to listen to what we had to say. Then he could have asked questions about the things he didn't understand and tried to give us insight as to what he thought. But we also knew we would have to make this decision for ourselves, not for them or anyone else.

Monday, I went home to Mom and Dad's for lunch with James. Phill warned me before I went that they would most likely say more that would make me cry, but I couldn't refuse to go home. The atmosphere wasn't tense at all, but over lunch, through the afternoon, and over supper, Mom and Dad kept talking to me and saying all kinds of things about the baby and our decision. They asked me hard questions that I felt I didn't have good enough answers for. So, mostly, I didn't give answers, just sat there and cried about how hopeless this decision was becoming.

On the way back to the city with James, I began to really think about what they had said, what my reasons were, and what would happen if we kept him. I realized that my resentment toward what they were saying wasn't right; it was rebellion and the opposite of keeping an open heart and mind.

I think the turning point was at James's apartment. He had to stop in to pick something up, and he invited me in to hear the newest song he had written. I sat there at his computer in the dark and listened to his voice singing what he had titled, "Paid For." It was a song about how Christians should live like they've been paid for by the blood of Jesus. I really thought about what that meant, and I decided that I shouldn't be living for myself. I shouldn't be making this decision for myself. I should be making it for God and for the baby. Both of them deserved my efforts. What better way is there to live my life?

During the evening, I was on the phone with lots of different people, including Leah and some of my friends. I tried to call Phill, but his phone was busy as well. I kept bouncing back and forth between placing the baby for adoption and parenting. I finally came to the conclusion, after all these months of trying to figure it out, that my only real reason for placing the baby was that I was too scared to keep him. That reason just wasn't good enough for me.

When I finally got through to Phill, he had talked to a bunch of people as well. His dad had called to apologize and tell him that he was impressed with how he had handled things. Phill had also talked to his brother Mark, who told him that kids and families are a gift that God blesses. He asked Phill if it were just up to him and there were no other people or their opinions involved, what would he do? Phill said he would keep our baby. Phill called my dad, too, and talked to him. The things these people told him made a lot of sense to him, he told me. He said that he agreed with them and thought we should go and get Joshua back. I felt the same way. Hearing him say it made my heart leap. It was strange how we changed our minds on our own and then just discovered that we thought the same way. But I think that was the miracle, all part of God's plan. So I called Leah right away and my parents next. I don't think my parents have cried so much in their lives as they have these past months. But, finally, I could give them a reason to cry tears of joy instead of sorrow, and I am so thankful for that.

After my phone calls were finished, I sat at my desk with thoughts of joy and wonder pouring through my mind. I looked at Karen sitting on her bed across from me and said, "I'm a mother. Someday I'm going to get Mother's Day gifts." The most precious of my thoughts was the realization that someday a little boy would start to call me "Mommy." Since the day I found out I was pregnant, I have never felt like a mother. Somehow I had convinced myself that I was having this baby for someone else, not for me. But in that one small moment in which Phill and I decided to change our minds, God handed me the ultimate gift: the privilege of becoming a mother. It was overwhelming to think about.

It is now Tuesday morning, and Keith and Lisa are bringing the baby to the city. Mom is picking me up to do some emergency baby shopping, then we're meeting at the agency with Phill, who is skipping school again, and getting our son. Our son. We've decided to name him Bailey Alexander.

Epilogue

Later that same day, my parents and I met Phill at the agency. While my parents waited in another room, Phill and I met with Keith and Lisa, who were holding our little boy. Without any kind of grudge or visible disappointment, they handed our baby to us and wished us luck. I can never thank them enough for being so understanding. When we entered the room where my parents sat and my dad saw us with our baby, he began to cry. Since that day, I don't believe I've ever known a happier, prouder grandpa.

Our lives changed drastically from then on. I quit my job and moved home with my parents. Phill quit university and bought me a big engagement ring. We were married in April and moved to his hometown, where our lives' ambition became taking over his dad's farm.

Our relationships with the other people in our lives gradually got better. Although we never sat down and resolved things with a lot of people who hurt us or whom we hurt, time healed us. In situations like ours, I believe that most times a person doesn't even realize they are hurting another by what they are doing or saying. Most of the people in our lives had never dealt with anything like this. They felt the need to say something but didn't know what to say, and often ended up saying something unintentionally hurtful even though they were trying to help. Realizing this has helped give us the ability to forgive and let go of whatever resentment we may have had.

One day not long after Bailey was born, Phill received a phone call on his cellphone from a girl in my church. Even though she didn't know Phill very well, she apologized to him for thinking badly of him during my pregnancy, though she had never said a word to him about it. Phill was touched by her apology and gained a deep respect for her because of her honesty and humility. I only wish that more of this kind of forgiveness could have taken place, instead of avoiding the subject and letting everything just blow over.

Although it hasn't been easy, we have never regretted our decision for a moment. We struggled with our physical relationship for the first year, perhaps because we had experienced too much of it before our wedding night. We didn't have any friends to go out with, since none of them lived close by and they were all still living a single's lifestyle. It was often frustrating that we couldn't just go out somewhere together because we had a baby to look after that we couldn't leave. But as it has always been between us, the difficulties made us stronger, and this time we turned to God for help. And help us He has. Our marriage has grown stronger and healthier.

Sometimes I wonder, how in the world did we get from being two troubled teenagers to being mature, stable parents? There is only one explanation, and that is because Jesus does wondrous things in our lives when we let Him. If we trust Him, He will do infinitely more than we can even imagine. I can't believe that even when I stopped looking to Him for guidance and made the decision without Him to place our baby, He still didn't abandon us. He made miracles happen. He took Phill's heart that didn't want marriage and didn't want children and turned it into a heart that asked me to marry him two weeks after Bailey's birth! He took my doubting and my impatience and my indecision and somehow got through to me, in that one moment at my brother's apartment, what I was supposed to do.

I certainly made mistakes along the way. The fact that we even made it through is a miracle in itself. Of all the things I did wrong,

I think the biggest one and the one that made all the difference was that I forgot, or refused, to listen to what Jesus was trying to tell me. Instead, I listened to other people around me and just dug my hole deeper. I could have saved myself a lot of grief by opening my heart to Him, regardless of what the other people in my life would say or do, and trusting Him to bring me through.

Some time after all of this happened, I attended a choir concert. One of the songs they sang really got through to me. I don't remember any of it except this one line: "He never failed me yet." At one time I used to wonder how people who wrote songs like this could really believe what they were writing. Could they really have that much faith and trust that they could sing such words? But now I know those words are true. He will never fail me, if I keep my hope and trust in Him. If you do the same, He will never fail you, either.

"I know we've been living like nothing's been given,
Getting madder when no one gives us more.
Would you change your ways in these scary days
When you figure out that we've been paid for?"[2]

Dear Journal,

Bailey is one month old today. It seems crazy that a whole month has gone by. Reading back in this journal is scary, seeing how close we came to giving our little boy away. As soon as we made the decision to keep him, I knew for certain we were doing the right thing. There was no doubt in my mind. And after I realized that, it was incredibly scary to read back on my thoughts from the months before. I don't exactly know what to make of all the things we thought.

I don't deserve any of this—I'm getting married, I have a beautiful fiancé and son, and the future looks bright. Everything has worked out wonderfully, and God has blessed us immensely. And what did we do? All we did was say one little word—"yes"—and this much has happened. What about all the selfishness, fear, distrust, and denial that went on for months? How does God possibly forget nine months of crap because of one second of righteousness? It amazes me how that works.

Endnotes

[1] Emilie Barnes, *15 Minutes Alone With God* (Oregon: Harvest House Publishing, 1994) pp. 27-29.

[2] Written by James Voth, "Paid For" 2001.

Resources

If you or someone you love is experiencing a crisis pregnancy, there are many Pregnancy Crisis Centres like the one I visited that are willing to help you. I encourage you to find one near you and talk to someone there about what you are thinking and feeling. Sometimes it helps just to talk. Centres also offer pregnancy tests, tons of literature and some offer abortion grief support. All services are confidential and free.

For more information or for a complete listing of Pregnancy Crisis Centres across Canada, visit the Canadian Association of Pregnancy Support Services Web site at www.capss.com. Or call the national toll free number 1-800-665-0570 to be referred to a centre near you.

In the US, please visit www.heartbeatinternational.org and click on the Worldwide Directory of Pregnancy Help to find a Pregnancy Crisis Centre near you or call the OptionLine help number listed on the site.